Teenagers: Growing Up and Sexuality

Dr. Carlos Ortiz Lee

Copyright © 2013 Carlos Ortiz Lee
All rights reserved.

To my parents, because they are the best of the world.

To my daughters Claudia, Patricia and Daniela
who make me see how beautiful life is.

To Elaine, for loving me so much.

ACKNOWLEDGMENTS

To "My Group," the ones that never stopped working for a moment. The ones that are always thinking of the future of adolescents and who continue to be my beloved colleagues of this specialty.

To all of you that contributed with me to complete this English version of my original book ¿Qué pasa en la adolescencia?

CONTENTS

Introduction / 11

The Body / 15

Female Genital Tract / 21

    Internal Genitals / 21

    External Genitals / 24

The Breasts / 33

Male Genital Tract / 41

    External Genitals / 41

    Internal Genitals / 46

Why Do These Changes Occur? / 49

    Other Changes / 51

Menstruation / 55

    Frequently Asked Questions / 61

    What About Hygiene? / 65

    The Calendar / 66

Ejaculation / 69

    Nocturnal Ejaculation / 71

Sexual Activity During Adolescence / 73

    Sex Without Intercourse / 76

    Masturbation / 80

    Anal Intercourse / 84

    When to Begin Having Intercourse? / 86

Pregnancy / 91
- For Girls / 91
- For Boys / 103
- For Both / 105

Contraceptive Methods / 107

Sexually Transmitted Diseases / 123

Your Friend the Gynecologist / 133

Epilogue / 135

INTRODUCTION

For us adults, this matter of adolescence can sometimes become a little complicated. Of course, for those of you who are just now beginning or finishing this beautiful stage of life, this is not so tangled, and you are feeling rather comfortable about this moment when you are becoming "grown up," and you are thinking that in so doing you will get out from under the constant orders that we parents are giving you children every minute. However, soon you will realize how fortunate you are that you will continue to be a "victim" of our orders for a while longer, although this may take you some time to understand.

I want to begin my explanations by speaking about the entire human body, which is much like the workings of a clock, and which, to function properly, needs all its pieces in good working order. But inside that great body "machine," which has so many organs working simultaneously, there are two that we can consider the most important: the brain and the heart.

The brain is the main organ of the central nervous system; it is like the great conductor of our body orchestra. Nothing happens in our body if it is not ordered by the brain.

Imagine how complete its mission is, that all these actions happen simultaneously. At this moment, for example, you are reading, but you have not stopped breathing. You can even start walking and yet continue to read while you walk. Still all the while your stomach is processing the last thing you ate, and your kidneys are making urine, which will make you go to the bathroom at any moment. So you can come to the conclusion that your brain spends twenty-four hours working and giving orders.

As you can imagine, this is not at all simple. The human body is made up of many organs and systems, each one with a different mission, and all —absolutely all— are directed and controlled by the brain.

In addition to the nervous system, which has an extensive network of nerves that run throughout the body and are in charge of carrying the messages transmitted by the brain, the other system with an organ essential to life is the cardiovascular system. The most important organ in this system is the heart. The heart starts to work many months before birth. Like the brain, it does not have one second to rest. It has to pump blood, in complete rhythm, throughout three hundred arteries and their branches in order to irrigate every centimeter of our bodies.

In short, one directs, and the other executes, but if one of the two fails, life ends —at least useful life. Without adequate brain function, it is impossible to sustain coordination or the necessary thought processes for a normal active life. However, independent of these vital systems, there are others that are no less important for sustaining life. These include the respiratory system, through which the lungs are in charge of oxygenating the blood, the digestive system, with its delicate and complicated job of processing nutrients from the moment we eat them, and other systems like the renal, auditory, visual, and musculoskeletal, which includes the bones, muscles, and joints. Finally, we get to the endocrine and the reproductive systems. The reproductive system will be the most discussed in this book. It is the one that is in charge of all the reproductive functions, including the production of many hormones that intervene in the functioning of the reproductive organs, including the genitals for both sexes. This complicated development process can last some four years.

The functional integration —that is to say, the coupling of all these organs and systems— is not at all simple, and they all work together intensely from birth (some even prior to birth) until death. Nevertheless, the changes occurring in the reproductive system during adolescence are very interesting, because they leave behind the image of the child in order to gradually transform us into men and women.

In a few years your body will go through so many changes that, by the end of your adolescence, it will seem to you that you are a different person. There is no other time in life that produces so many modifications so quickly, as in this stage.

To help you better understand your body, I will refer to some of these important changes that occur in the body with more detail later —for example, changes in the genital tracts of both sexes. We will also review some interesting questions about their function.

THE BODY

Adolescence is a beautiful time of life during which we start to leave childhood behind in order to start a complicated biological process that will transform us into adults. However, it takes ten years from the time we are born to arrive at adolescence. The body takes advantage of these years to grow and develop the different organs.

The daily language of pediatricians, doctors who specialize in children, always includes the words "growth and development," precisely because they reflect in great measure the quality of life for each of us during the first few years of life. These are the two most important aspects associated with well-being during our childhood: we grow, and our bodies continue to develop. If you remember your visits to the doctor when you were little, generally the first things the doctor did was weigh you and measure you. Oftentimes, the results of those measurements were enough to alert your parents about something that was irregular. The process of interrupted growth or development is determined by many factors. Some are out of our control, and we cannot modify them, like genetic influences that we inherit from our parents. Some that are no less important, like nutrition, exercise, proper sleep, among others, depend to a great extent on us and therefore can be modified.

I believe you will find it interesting to know that studies about growth and development exist on a national level in many countries, and that research has established standards that guide doctors regarding these issues.

If a child measures or weighs, or both, over or under the limits established as average according to these standards, the child should submit to more tests without delay. The growth and development of a child with proper nutrition as well as reasonable parameters of physical activity, sleep, and adequate education for his or her age, will not be the same as the development of a child for whom any of these factors are abnormal, either because the child is excessive or lacking.

We all know, for example, if nutrition is insufficient, growth and development will be below normal limits. In the case of excessive nutrition or poor quality nutrition, the results will not be very encouraging either. In those cases normal development will be threatened by a worldwide silent enemy of this modern era: childhood obesity.

Sadly, only very few people are aware that obesity is not a condition but an illness whose consequences are very dangerous over time and for which prevention is a much better alternative than treatment.

I am not going to bore you with long explanations about growth during infancy; you are probably not interested in learning about that subject, since you have already gone beyond that stage. So it is better for us to concentrate on some issues more closely related to adolescence, which will be with you for several years.

After infancy is over, this process of growth and development does not stop, but it is at this time that it acquires a peculiarity that distinguishes it from childhood: the influence of the hormones, which are the real players of this phase. During this period many changes happen in our bodies. All the organs and systems that comprise it participate in one way or another, and it is due to the actions of the hormones that these changes can happen.

Hormones are chemical substances produced by specific organs, and they are capable of unleashing actions in others. The bones elongate and become harder. The muscles develop more. We grow at a much faster rate than we did during childhood. Our voice tone changes, and simultaneously, important changes appear in the organs of our reproductive system that prepare them for having children. Certain parts of these modifications are not appreciated by you, but others are. In this way, the body progressively changes during this magical time in which our hormones begin to wake up after a long sleep, and this happens just when the brain has to start working with more intensity, because it must handle an increasing learning load in school. At the same time, it has to continue to take care of the body's other functions without taking a vacation.

When do these changes start? Well, the answer cannot be categorical, because biology does not allow rigidity. This means that these changes are progressive and individual. In other words, they happen bit by bit and in a different way from one adolescent to another. That is why they can begin at different ages for each adolescent. For example, some young women begin to menstruate when they are nine years old, and others may have to wait until they are fourteen or fifteen. In boys, the changes of puberty may happen earlier for some than for others.

If you could think right now about your friends from school, especially those you have known since you were little, you would be able to see that some are shorter and some taller, some chubbier and others more slender.

Teenagers: growing up and sexuality

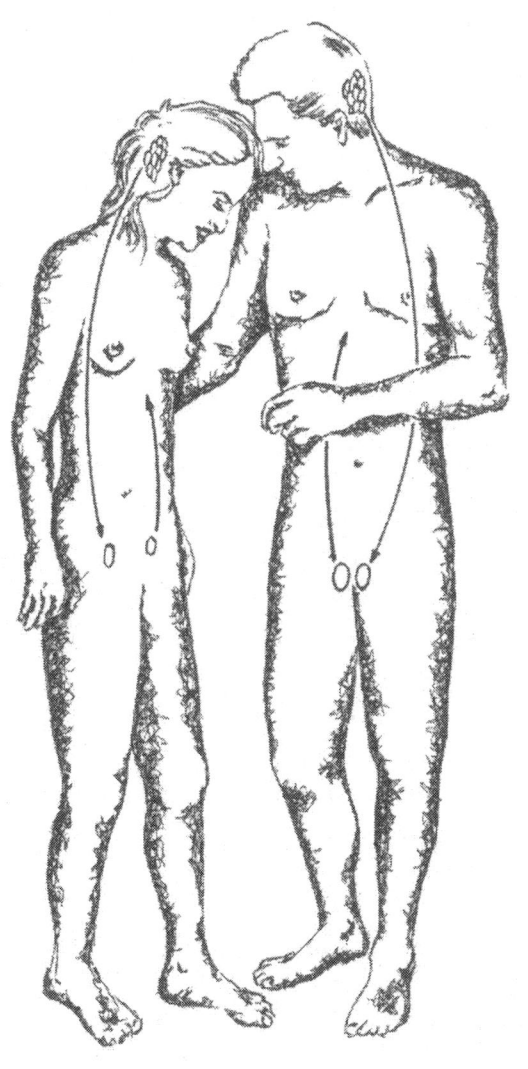

The exact thing happens with the changes that occur inside your body, so that "development," as it is sometimes called, can in some cases, begin earlier than in others.

No matter which way or at what age it occurs, adolescence begins this process that will fill you with questions. We are going to review some aspects of the anatomy of the reproductive apparatus, and later we will review some of the issues about this interesting time of life.

FEMALE GENITAL TRACT

The female genital tract is made up of various organs and structures, some of which are located in the interior of the abdomen, specifically in the lowest part, and some of which are perfectly visible, since they are located externally.

As you can see in the illustration, all the organs are different from each other, since each one has a specific function. However, all the organs are equally important, because their work is very interrelated, and many times the function of one organ depends totally on what another has done. In other words, it is truly teamwork. For example, if the ovaries do not produce an ovum, an egg, as you will see shortly, the uterus cannot develop a pregnancy.

Internal Genitals

Among the internal genitals of the female reproductive tract is the uterus, which measures 7 to 8 cm in length and 4 to 5 cm in width, can weigh up to 100 g, and is located in the center of the female pelvis. So you can better imagine it, I will tell you that it is shaped like a pear and that it is divided into two parts: the body and the neck.

The body of the uterus fits totally inside the abdominal cavity, in a location that many people call the "lower abdomen," while the neck projects toward the vagina and is the only part that a doctor can see when he does a gynecological examination.

The uterus is an important organ, because it is where pregnancy develops, and that is its specific function in the female body. It is made up of a very powerful muscular mass that allows it to greatly increase its size while the future baby develops inside of the uterus, where it will be maintained during the entire pregnancy.

It can stretch so much, that at times pregnancies of twins or triplets, the uterus is capable of continued growth so that the babies can all fit in that warm "home" in which we live for a few months before birth.

In addition to the uterus, right there inside the abdomen are the ovaries and the fallopian tubes. In contrast to the uterus, which is only one organ, the ovaries, as well as the fallopian tubes, are duplicated and situated on each side of the uterus, with which they communicate directly.

The ovaries are much smaller than the uterus. They measure 3 to 5 cm in length, 1.5 to 3 cm in width, about 0.5 to 1.5 cm thick, and they are shaped precisely like an egg.

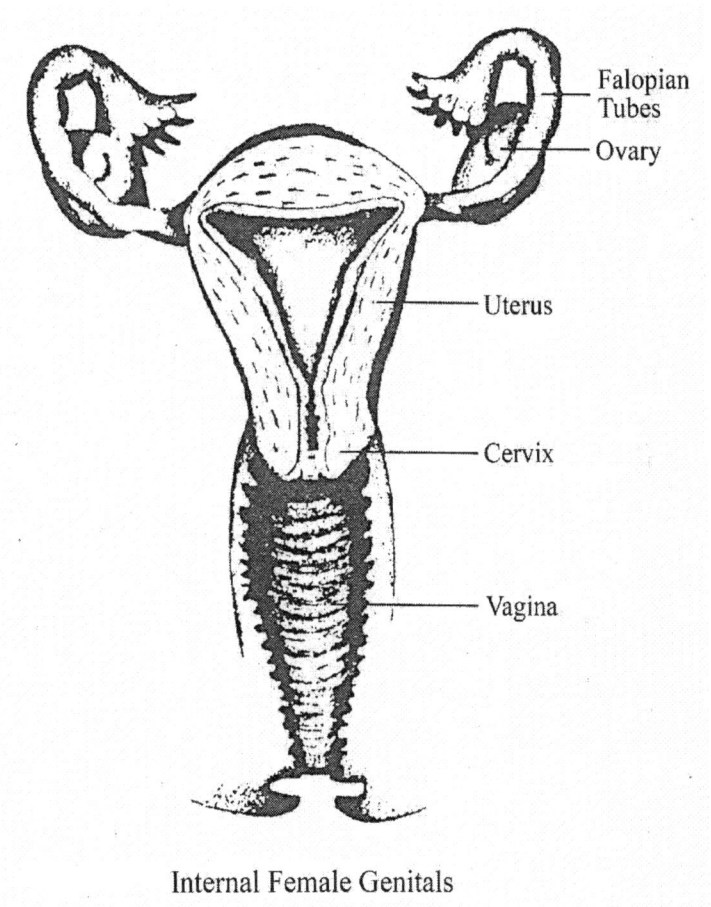

Internal Female Genitals

Small structures called follicles are located inside the ovaries, and they contain the ovum, the female reproductive cell. The ovum is so small that it cannot be seen with the naked eye. So you have an idea, I will tell you that the size of one ovum is approximately one-tenth of a millimeter. Tiny, right?

The ovaries are very important to a woman's health, because of the function they perform, which will be explained later in more detail.

The fallopian tubes, for their part, are like two little hoses, the longest of which can reach up to 12 cm in length. They are not solid: they have an internal open duct throughout their entire length that connects to the uterus at one end and is open to the abdominal cavity on the other.

These are the female organs that are inside the abdomen. Now that you know them better, I will explain something about the other ones, the ones you can easily observe.

External Genitalia

The vulva is situated between the Venus mount, which is the area that in these years of adolescence will begin to be covered by pubic hair, and the anus.

On both sides of the vulva, you can see some folds of skin that are small at first and, as you begin to grow, become thicker. These are called the labia majora. Inside these, there are other, smaller, folds of skin. Those are the labia minora.

I want to pause a moment here to make a comment about the labia minora.

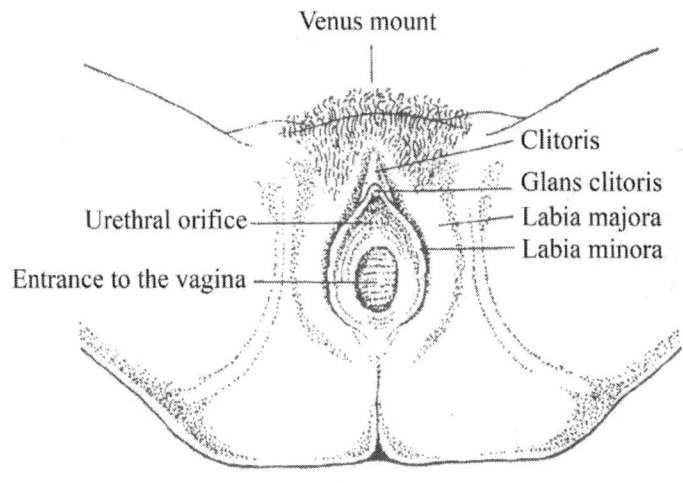

External Female Genitalia

As their name indicates, these are smaller than the labia majora. However, I can tell you that, although the great majority of young women fall inside this norm, there are some young women who experience more development of these tissues.

In such cases, these may protrude more than usual, so if this is the case with you, know that there is no cause for alarm.

In spite of this, I can tell you that in my practice, I saw with relative frequency, adolescents and also adult women, who were so very worried about the volume of their labia minora.

Occasionally, some even insisted on executing surgical procedures in order to reduce them, due to discomfort. However, in the great majority of these cases, these patients wanted surgical reduction only on the basis that they considered them unattractive.

There are exceptional cases where an operation to reduce the size of the labia minora could be considered, however, surgery is usually not recommended, because it can cause great discomfort due to shrinking of the skin, which would affect the anatomy and sensitivity of those tissues.

Just at the top of the vulva, where the labia minora come together, is the clitoris. It is approximately the same size as a pencil eraser and is very sensitive to the touch. During sexual contact, brushing against this zone produces very pleasing sensations for the woman. Under the clitoris, also in the center, there is a small orifice, called the external urethral orifice, through which urine comes out. It is not part of the genital tract, but I mention it because it is situated in that area.

If the labia are separated, just at the entrance to the vagina, one can see a thin membrane called the *hymen*, which can vary in form.

For this reason it can be called different names, as you see in the illustration. It has a minimum of one orifice, but can have various ones, and it is through these that the blood from menstruation comes through.

It is good for you to know that the hymen will not accompany women throughout their lifetime, as it usually disappears once sexual relations are initiated. Occasionally, it does not disappear completely until after the first birth delivery.

Many years ago, the presence of the hymen was like a letter of introduction for young women who were headed for matrimony since it signified that they were "virgins" that is, that they had never participated in the sexual act.

All this because in those times women were prohibited from having sexual intercourse until after they were married, and those women who did not abstain in that manner were classified as women without honor.

Back then, people did many things, which are hard for us to believe today, in order to ensure that the newly married woman had in fact been a virgin until her wedding night.

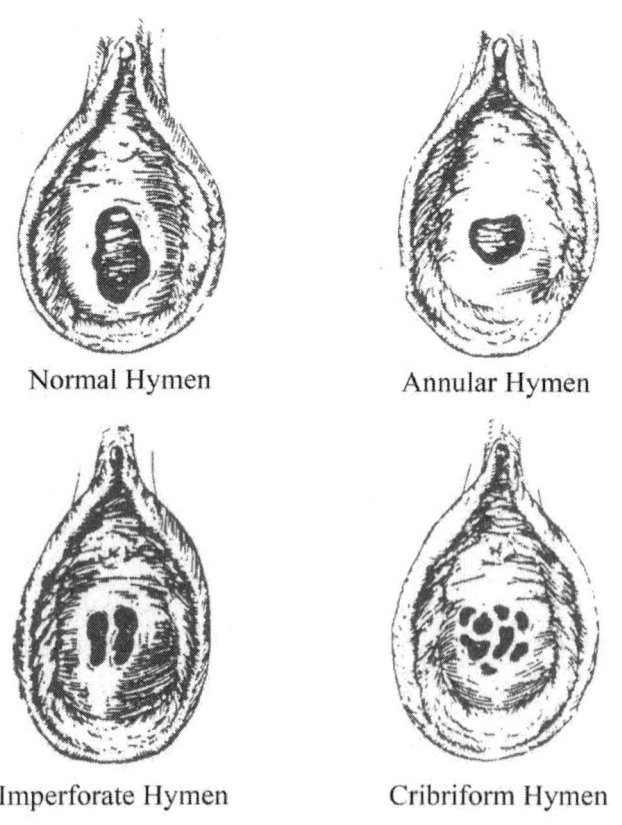

Types of Hymen

In many places, people went to the extreme of waiting by the door of the just-married couple's bedroom for the groom to show the sheet with the bloody mark sometimes produced during the first sexual contact as a result of the torn hymen.

This is an example, of many that exist, of the discrimination that women have suffered throughout the centuries, since at no time have there been any such requirements imposed upon men regarding marriage and their virginity.

Luckily, except for some isolated cultures, this absurd way of evaluating the honor of women no longer exists. Because, in actuality, in most of the civilized world, it does not matter if young ladies retain their improperly named "virginity" until their wedding night. Besides, the hymen is a membrane which has certain elasticity, and due to that fact, there are many times when it produces absolutely no bleeding during the first sexual intercourse.

Imagine what awaited those who could not demonstrate the famous bloody stain on the sheets! Fortunately, as I was telling you, those prejudices from our grandparents have gradually disappeared.

In some places, people overvalue an intact hymen to the point that they forbid adolescent women to use vaginal tablets and tampons.

It is good for you to know that the majority of adolescents can use tampons during their menstrual periods without any difficulty, even if they have never had sexual intercourse. Nor will they have any impediment using a vaginal tablet treatment if they should ever develop a vaginal infection, since the elasticity of the hymen allows it without any damage, not only in adolescents but also in younger girls.

During my medical practice, I have personally treated many adolescents and girls with chronic vaginal infections that were effectively healed with the use of vaginal tablets. The problem of insertion is resolved very easily by teaching the parents, or even the girls, how to correctly insert the tablets.

I want to be very clear on this: the use of tampons or vaginal tables has no relationship whatsoever to the supposed loss of virginity.

The vagina, for its part, is long and moist. It can measure up to 10 cm and has rough inner walls that are dense but very elastic. This allows the interior to receive the penis during sexual intercourse and to let the baby pass through during birth. That elasticity of the vagina also allows the gynecologist to use the speculum during medical examinations.

Before going on, I will explain what the speculum is and what it is used for. Because it has such a strange name, like all the names that doctors invent, you may not even have heard about it, and I do not want you to have any doubts.

The speculum is a small instrument with two valves, or parts, that the doctor softly introduces into the vagina to observe every side of the walls of the vagina and the neck of the uterus. We used to call that part of the uterus "the cervix".

This serves to detect many conditions in those areas; to introduce or remove contraceptive devices that are placed inside the uterus; and to do Pap smears, a very important test for all women during their adult lives.

A Pap smear is a simple test, which does not hurt at all, that is done to detect pre-cancerous lesions in the neck of the uterus.

It is important for you to know this, because this test can discover these conditions early, which gives us the opportunity to treat them completely with a variety of treatments, many times even without the need for surgery.

If you ask your mom, she can tell you about her experiences with this simple and, at the same time, necessary procedure.

THE BREASTS

The mammaries, or breasts, —you can call them by what name you prefer— also begin to grow in adolescence.

During all of childhood, there is no visible difference in a boy's upper body when we compare it to a girl's body. But during adolescence or puberty, girls will begin to develop mammary glands (that is what breasts are called), and little by little, they will begin to change. Most of the time, this is the first change that girls notice about their bodies, and it happens even before they have their first period or first menstruation. This is when everything turns into an event, because it represents the first big change in a girl's body that can be seen through her clothes.

The first thing that happens is the increase in the volume of the nipple and areola, which is the zone of darker skin that surrounds the nipple. Later, little by little, the volume of the breast increases in a way that the fatty tissue that forms it begins to develop until it reaches its definitive size, which varies with each adolescent girl, depending on a diversity of factors.

One important detail to keep in mind is that the breasts sometimes may not begin their development simultaneously, but that development may begin in one first and the other later. This is completely normal, and if it happens to you, do not worry about it at all. With the passage of time, by the end of adolescence, they will reach a similar look and size, although it is relatively common to find that one breast will be discretely larger than the other. This difference many times is not noticeable. This is normal, so you should not worry if this happens to you or to some of your friends.

In some cases, when this growth and development are taking place in the breasts, you can feel some sensation of discomfort that sometimes can even be slightly painful, and this is part of the normal physical process. It normally disappears in a short time without treatment, for which reason it does not require too much of our attention.

I want to make a comment about something else here, and that is about size, because breasts come in different shapes and sizes, like you have probably noticed by observing the women around you. These differences are not important either. This means that when adolescence is over, some young women will have big and voluptuous breasts that will grow toward the front and be very firm, others will have breasts that are inclined downward, and yet another group will have small breasts.

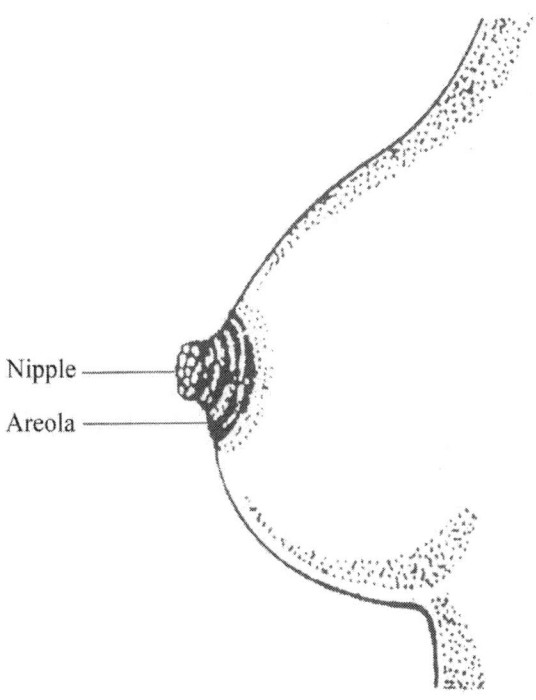

Parts of the Breast

All these varieties are normal, and it is very important that you know this, because sometimes young women worry about the size or shape of the breasts, and that has nothing whatsoever to do with what happens when it is time to nurse a baby.

The growth of the breasts depends on the amount of fatty tissue that is deposited in them, and that does not affect the glandular tissues at all, which is the part that is important for the function of nursing the baby.

Besides, the size of the breasts is not important for sexual relations either, since sensations of pleasure experienced with petting, stroking, or brushing against the breasts is absolutely not related at all to their size or form.

What is important for that are the nerve endings, which are the ones that provoke excitement when they are stimulated. Those nerve endings have the same capacity of reaction for all the varieties that exist, independent of the size and the shape of the breasts.

With this clarification, if you are part of the group that has small breasts, you should now have less worry in your life. In the same way that some of your male friends like chubby girls and others like slender girls, some will be more attracted to girls with voluptuous breasts and the rest to girls with small breasts. With breasts that are inclined downward, it seems to be a bit different because they are mistakenly associated with the physical drooping that occurs with the passing of time and, sincerely, there is no reason to look at it that way.

Sometimes the breasts turn downward since the beginning of their development and retain that form at the end of adolescence. That is also normal.

Remember that tastes vary a lot. Therefore, the size and shape of your breasts should not be, in any way, a reason to worry.

In any case, when you have any doubt in relation to the development, the volume, or the shape of your breasts, it is recommended that you visit your gynecologist. After a detailed physical examination, the doctor is the only one who can give you the guidance regarding your development and reproductive health concerns. I tell you this because a lot of times, patients will resort to operative procedures for either implants for breast enlargement, or reductions for excessively large breasts.

Personally I do not support either option. During my experiences in a vast number of operating rooms, I have seen many surgical complications that could have been prevented or avoided altogether. So my advice is to go into an operating room only when it is absolutely necessary. For those girls who have such small breasts that they want to experiment with hormone treatments, I also say to them that I do not recommend it, since to this day no treatment has demonstrated any effect in successfully attaining the desired increase in size.

The underdevelopment of the breasts is associated with reduced activity of the estrogen receptors in the breasts. Therefore exogenous estrogen will not have any significant effect if receptor activity is the underlying problem. Furthermore administering estrogen to an adolescent who does not need it may cause more harm than good.

I have already mentioned some interesting issues about the growth and development of the breasts in this chapter, but I am not going to end it without mentioning a tremendously important aspect of it: the self-examination of the breasts.

In females, illnesses related to the breasts are relatively common, from congenital malformations (that is, those that are present at birth) to tumors of various origins, all the way to the most worrisome of all: breast cancer. This disease costs thousands of women of all ages their lives every day.

All young women should know how to perform this self-examination. For proper instructions, she should visit, at the earliest opportunity, her primary physician or gynecologist, who will be very happy to explain it.

When women get used to performing this monthly self-examination of the breasts, it will be very difficult for them to miss any irregularity that may present itself, be it a painful mass, a hardening, a simple little "ball," or a discoloration of the skin.

With this simple examination, women can discover the most minimal alteration that may appear. In spite of this, there are still some who do not want to do the self-exam and others who, when they find an abnormality, refuse to visit the doctor. This is a mistake: the sooner you can detect some change, the better the possibility of a complete cure. It is precisely this quick action that can avoid a big operation. And even if a mastectomy (removal of the breast) is required, reconstructive surgery will restore a normal, natural appearance.

It is true that breast cancer continues to be frequent in women, but it is also true that by performing a monthly self-examination of the breasts and consulting a specialist at the first sign of a change, the outcome can be much better, and breast cancer deaths can be avoided.

Fortunately, breast cancer is really rare during adolescence. During this time of life, benign illnesses are more common. These can also usually be discovered with a simple examination of the breast and can be treated with great success once diagnosed.

These changes may appear, as previously stated, as a hard little ball on a breast. It doesn't hurt and can easily move when you touch it. This is a characteristic of benign nodules, which represents approximately 95 percent of all tumors of the breast that are removed in adolescence. Surgery is done by making a small incision in the affected breast and taking out the nodule, and the problem is usually resolved.

Other times, instead of finding a nodule, you will feel a discomfort in the breasts that can turn into painful episodes. Sometimes this happens during menstruation, and in these cases the cause of this discomfort is related to normal changes in hormone levels. Generally, these discomforts are temporary; they have to do with the development of the breasts and do not require medical treatment.

In any case, when you have any worry about your breasts, be it their size, pain, or for any other reason, you should always reach out to a gynecologist, who will examine you and guide you regarding what you should do.

MALE GENITAL TRACT

The organs of the male reproductive system are also divided into external and internal, according to their location. Their proper functioning is indispensable for the reproductive life of men.

External Genitalia

The penis is an organ that is made up of cylindrical structures, as you can see in the illustration: they are the corpora cavernosa, which are located in the upper part, one next to the other, and, underneath these, the corpus spongiosum.

The corpora cavernosa cover the entire area of the penis, and through each of them passes an important artery that fills them with blood.

At the time of sexual arousal, the volume of blood increases in these arteries inside the corpora cavernosa, and this is what contributes to a penile erection, as well as the increase in dimension, since the penis becomes bigger when erect.

At the anterior end of the penis is the *glans* or the *head*, which is an area that is very sensitive to the touch. It is made up of many nerve endings. Because of this, the slightest touch during sexual activity unleashes pleasurable sensations.

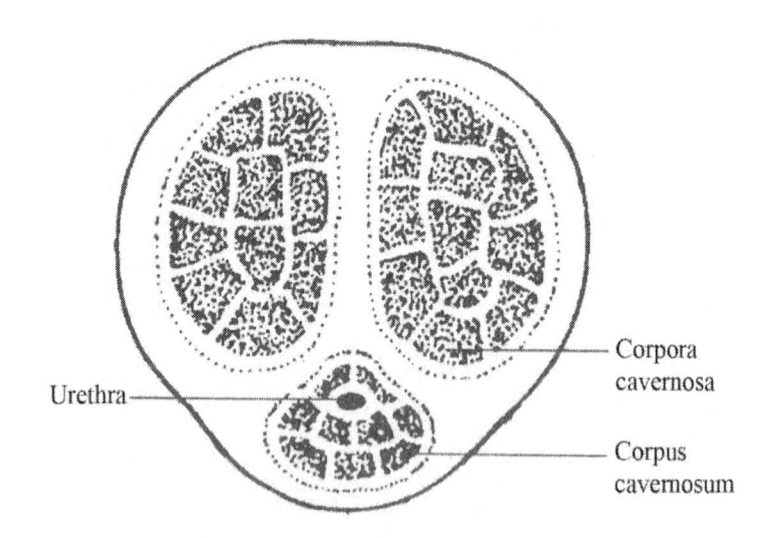

Transverse section of the penis

The skin that covers the *glans* is called *prepuce*. It is retractable: that is, it can be pulled back by hand, leaving the glans uncovered. It is normal to be able to slide the foreskin back without difficulty, however, sometimes this can cause some pain, and the skin may not be totally retractable. In these cases it is necessary to perform a simple surgical procedure called circumcision, which involves removing the prepuce.

Phimosis, which is the scientific name for this condition, may occur due to a narrowing of the opening of the prepuce. This condition is diagnosed with relative frequency during childhood. At times, it can also be present in adult males as a result of local infections due to the accumulation of the normal secretions produced in this area between the glans and the prepuce. (Notice that I am speaking in the same language that doctors use, because it is the best way for you to really understand these concepts. If I say to you "the foreskin," as the prepuce is commonly called, maybe my explanation will not sound very serious.) This infection causes local irritation and inflammation, and can not only lead to phimosis, but it is also a favorable condition for the onset of cancer of the penis in later years. This makes genital hygiene very important in order to avoid these complications.

It is good for you to know that circumcision is not only done to treat phimosis; in some cultures and countries, the surgical stripping of the prepuce is done in bulk and for various reasons, including cultural or religious. So, if you have been circumcised, or if you have noticed that some of your friends have had this procedure, it does not mean that they have had phimosis.

Another important aspect in the anatomy of the penis is its external appearance. Two very well-known sexologists, Masters and Johnson, wrote a book called *Human Sexuality*, which in one of its chapters states, "It is not much of an exaggeration to say that penises in fantasyland come in only three sizes —large, gigantic, and so big you can barely get them through the doorway," and that is because there are all kinds of legends relating sexual potency to the size of the penis. I can tell you that there is nothing further from the truth.

As I pointed out in another chapter, if you notice your classmates, you can be sure that they are all different in height: some are tall, some short, some heavier, and some skinnier. The size of the penis happens in the exact same way. Some will have bigger dimensions than others. However, one particular factor makes them different, and that is that in the moment of sexual arousal. Whereas the smallest penis can double in size, the biggest ones, when erect, only increase in length by a small increment. For this reason, young men should absolutely not worry about the size of their penises. In addition, the walls of the vagina, like I explained before, are normally close together, and when the penis is inserted, they adapt to any size without having any difficulty feeling the pleasurable sensations that a couple experiences during coital relations.

Besides the penis, externally, you can also see the scrotum. This is the bag inside which you can find the testicles. The skin of the scrotum is wrinkled and darker than that of the abdomen, and it is less sensitive than the skin of the glans —although touching the scrotum can also produce pleasurable sensations during mutual caressing.

Lastly there is the urethra, which is the duct through which the semen and urine flow and which is between 20 and 23 cm in length. The urethra is a little of both, internal and external genitalia, because it begins in the bladder, travels through the prostate, and continues to the penis, ending its long journey at the glans, where you can see the external *urethral orifice*. This is the little hole that we can all see at the end of the penis.

In boys, the urethra is important for reproductive function. Besides being the duct through which urine is excreted, like I said before, it is also the duct through which sperm is released.

At this time you are probably asking if it is possible for the sperm and the urine to come out through the urethra at the same time. Well, the answer to that question is no.

Remember that the human body is an almost perfect machine —more so than even modern computers— and when ejaculation is about to happen, the urethra automatically closes at the end where the urine comes into it. It does this so that the sperm cannot get into the bladder or the urine into the urethra.

Internal Genitalia

Among the organs that you cannot see from outside are the testicles. These are the glands that, in adults, are approximately 4 cm long, 3 cm wide and 2 cm thick. They are very important in the development of the reproductive life of boys, since they are responsible for the production of male hormones and the development of sperm. The testicles produce androgens, which are principally responsible for the changes that occur in the genital tracts of boys. The end result is an increase in the size of the scrotum and the testicles.

Testosterone is the hormone that is responsible for the modifications that differentiate boys from girls. It also initiates enlargement of the larynx, one of the respiratory organs, which brings about the change from a child's voice to a man's voice, among other important functions.

The production of sperm also starts during puberty, and once it starts, it does not rest. It is estimated that thousands of millions of sperm are generated per year. This process takes place in a few small structures, which doctors have given one of those strange names that they give to the parts of our bodies: *seminiferous tubules.*

Internally, there is also a large, thin, elongated structure called *epididymis.* It extends all the way along the back of each testicle, to which it is connected at one end. The other end is connected to the *vas deferens.*

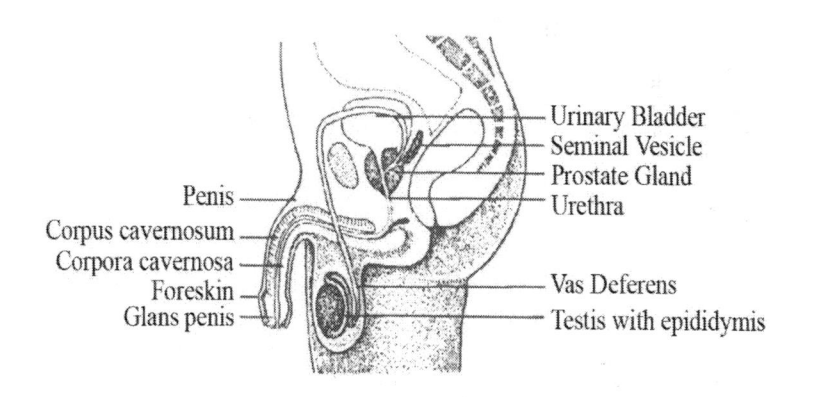

Transverse section of the male genitals

At the entrance of the urethra, there are two other structures: the *seminal vesicle* and the *prostate.*

There are two *seminal vesicles*. They are located above the prostate, and each is joined to its corresponding vas deferens, forming the ejaculatory duct, through which the sperm travel on their way out. I am complicating somewhat this little tour of the male genitalia, but if you look carefully at the illustrations it will be much easier for you to locate everything.

The *prostate* is just under the bladder, and it weighs around 20 g. Another portion of the urethra, which as I told you is pretty long, also traverses through it.

Under the prostate there are some small glands that during sexual arousal, just before ejaculation, secrete a few drops of fluid that serve to eliminate the acidic residue of urine from the urethra in order to protect the sperm. These secretions also travel through the urethra. This secretion comes out through the external orifice of the penis, and even though it is not yet time for ejaculation, it usually contains a small amount of sperm.

This is very important to know, because it is one of the reasons that *coitus interruptus* fails as a method of birth control. I will explain about this variance when we talk about the different methods of birth control.

WHY DO THESE CHANGES OCCUR?

The functioning of the different organs that compose our body depends on a complex series of events that are all directed by the brain.

There is a small gland located in the brain called the *pituitary gland* that directs and controls the functions of other glands. Among these glands are the gonads —that is, the ovaries and the testicles.

A hormone is produced in the female pituitary and transported throughout the body in the bloodstream. This hormone, for its part, initiates the secretion of the hormones that are produced by the ovaries.

Out of all the organs in the female reproductive system, the ovaries work the hardest. In the early stages of puberty, the brain gives the ovaries an order to begin producing hormones. In this case, these hormones are the *estrogens,* which influence, in one way or another, all of the female body. Although the ovaries are their principal fountain of production, estrogens also have a lot to do with the development of other organs unrelated to the reproductive system.

In summary, we can say that this hormonal secretion carries most of the responsibility for the development of what we call female sexual characteristics.

Thanks to the direct or indirect work of these hormones and others no less important, young women will experience many changes during adolescence. Their voices will change, becoming more acute, and their hips will become wider and their buttocks more voluminous.

In the female genital tract, estrogens stimulate the development of all the organs, with the objective of completing their formation. They are also responsible for the growth and development of the breasts, preparing them for lactation with the help of another hormone.

For boys, there is also a hormonal stimulus from this small structure called the pituitary gland that will take the message to the testicles. The testicles are responsible for changes in the boy's body through the progressive synthesis of *androgens*. These hormones are the male version of what estrogens are for girls. In a few years, as a result of the hormonal secretions of the testicles, men can reproduce. This is all in addition to the external changes previously mentioned.

Other Changes

In conjunction with the previously mentioned hormones, other hormones contribute to the changes in the body during adolescence. During this time, changes happen throughout the entire body, not just to the reproductive system. The changes that are taking place in the reproductive system during this phase are so striking and so exciting that sometimes we think they are the only important changes that occur during puberty. Not at all!

The growth hormones, for example, also produced by the pituitary, have a determining role in the final stature that you will attain as an adult. In adolescence the familiar "growth spurt" is generated. During this time we grow much more rapidly than in childhood. In girls it usually happens between the ages of eleven and twelve, while in boys it begins between twelve and fifteen years of age. This explains why a lot of times girls are taller than boys at this age. However, approximately around 14 years of age, the boys will grow more than the girls and will end up being taller by an average of 12 to 13 cm at the end of adolescence.

It is difficult to predict the rate of growth for each individual person. Keeping this in mind, all these numbers and data given here may vary, because so many different elements influence this process.

In any case, the workload for the body at this time is huge. Imagine how hard the different organs of the body have to work once this growth spurt happens. It is not the same for the heart, for example, to pump enough blood to irrigate the small body of a child as that of an adolescent who is twice the size and of course weighs more. And this development is happening throughout the entire body.

Most of the changes experienced during adolescence are welcome by young people. These changes signify that they are, all of a sudden, turning into men and women, and this makes them happy, since we all want to be "big." However, during puberty, sometimes there are other transitional changes, unexpected by young people, that may be unpleasant. Sometimes these changes cause situational conflicts due to self-esteem issues, which are baseless but very annoying to those who are going through them. Among these unwanted phenomena, for example, are acne and goiter, big enemies of adolescents.

Acne is an inflammatory infection of the skin produced by a combination of hormonal and genetic factors that appears with varying intensity in up to 80 to 90 percent of adolescents. It is characterized by the presence of skin lesions and excessive accumulation of oils in blocked pores on the cheeks, and in a smaller number of cases it can be seen on the forehead, chin, neck, and chest. Luckily, acne is temporary and usually disappears spontaneously at the end of adolescence. In some young people it can continue for a longer period of time and can even cause local infections that require medical attention. Even though the causes for these infections are benign, it is important to see the doctor in order to receive instructions about how to eliminate the problem. Treatment may vary according to sex or even among adolescents of the same sex. I believe that it is important for you to know, this since the doctor is always the best person to guide you toward an adequate resolution of your problem. It is important to avoid self-treatment, because in many cases it may not resolve the problem, and may be a waste of time and money with unpleasant consequences.

In the case of goiter, you should know that, during adolescence an increase in the size of the thyroid gland may appear. This is due to the excessive activity to which this gland is subjected during puberty. The thyroid is located exactly in the front of the neck, and this condition is more frequent in girls than boys. In adolescents with goiter, you can see an increased volume to the front of the neck that is not only visible, but palpable, and which generally has no health implication. It usually disappears spontaneously at the end of adolescence. In any case, when this happens, a visit to the doctor is recommended to determine if the goiter is, in fact, related to puberty, or if it is due to another cause that should be identified and treated. This is important, because sometimes the cause of the goiter is something else that, if not discovered and treated promptly, can result in bigger health problems.

In addition to all these changes that I have mentioned so far, in adolescence there are two very important events which mark milestones in the development of human beings: menstruation in girls and ejaculation in boys. The following chapters are dedicated to these interesting processes.

MENSTRUATION

For many years, menstruation was a forbidden subject. We just didn't talk about it. For this reason, adolescent girls had their menarche (the name that has been given to the first menstruation) without having the slightest idea what was happening in their bodies.

If you talk with your mother and your grandmothers, you can confirm what I am telling you. Many of them were scared when faced with the first menstrual bleeding, thinking that they had a wound, or that they had some inexplicable illness. Usually someone would tell them that was their "period" or "time of the month," and just like that, without any more information they began to wait each month for their menstruation.

Fortunately, with the passage of time, this mistaken practice has gradually changed, and today it is pretty hard for a girl to arrive at this moment of her life with such minimal information. In spite of this fact, we can still find some families who prefer to continue to act in an antiquated manner. And what happens in those cases is that girls find out what they want to learn or need to learn through their friends at school.

The first menstruation is a very important event in the life of an adolescent, since it always arrives with many questions. So, what is menstruation? How does it happen?

During adolescence, the organs of the reproductive system are getting prepared for the future, for when the moment arrives to have children. In the case of girls, the establishment of the menstrual cycle is a signal that indicates that the female genital tract is well developed.

The brain —again with the brain— starts to give new orders so that the internal organs of the female reproductive system will start to function. In this sense, the first step it takes is to put to work some hormones that have to do with that area of the body. This stimulates the work of the ovaries, with the goal of bringing one of the follicles it contains to maturity, so that it can release one of the eggs inside it.

At the same time, the fallopian tubes are put on alert in order to attract the ovum (egg) when it is released from the follicle and draw it into its inner channel. There the ovum waits for the arrival of the sperm (masculine reproductive cell) with the objective of producing fertilization.

Once an egg is fertilize, which happens inside the fallopian tube, the brain continues to emit signals. These signals prepare the uterus to receive the previously fertilized ovum. The pregnancy cannot develop in the fallopian tube, because it is very narrow; therefore the place intended for that purpose is the uterus, because of its great capacity to expand.

There is so much happening that the first thing that comes to mind is a question: How do they manage to do all that? Well, first the follicle in one of the ovaries breaks, and the egg comes out of that follicle. In that very moment, the fallopian tube attracts the follicle as if it was a magnet and transports it through its inner channel. Once there, it detains the follicle and makes it wait for a while. But why wait in such a narrow place? The problem is that the ovum by itself is not enough to produce a pregnancy, and since the objective of this whole process is reproduction, the egg must wait patiently for its encounter with the sperm in order to produce fertilization.

How does sperm get up there? During sexual intercourse, with the insertion of the penis into the vagina, the semen (fluid containing the sperm) is deposited in the vagina near the entrance to the neck of the uterus. This means that sperm have to travel a great distance in order to reach the ovum and fertilize it. Although this really seems very complicated for all of us, the sperm resolve it very easily, thanks to their great mobility.

Of course, adolescence is not the season for pregnancy, and since the ovaries know this, sometimes they do not even let the follicles break. Because of this, adolescent girls will go through several months without ovulating, which is what the process is called.

Pregnancy is for adulthood, because during adolescence, as you will see later, pregnancy has many risks.

Once ovulation occurs, the estrogens, which are joined at this time by another hormone called progesterone, are responsible for preparing the uterus to receive the egg, fertilized or not fertilized. This leads to the formation of a rather thick layer, which rests against the interior wall of the uterus, called endometrium.

If the ovum is fertilized, which is what will happen when you decide to have children, then the pregnancy will start to develop inside the uterus. However, if there is no fertilization, the ovum, along with the thick layer that has formed, will separate from the uterine wall and leave the body through the vagina. This is what we call *menstruation*. From this point on, the brain again orders the follicle to mature, and this cycle repeats itself, again and again, bringing on the onset of menstruation every month. However, when a pregnancy is produced, menstruation disappears until after childbirth.

The reason this happens is precisely what I explained, that menstruation is the shedding of the endometrial lining that forms in the second half of the menstrual cycle, influenced by estrogen and progesterone.

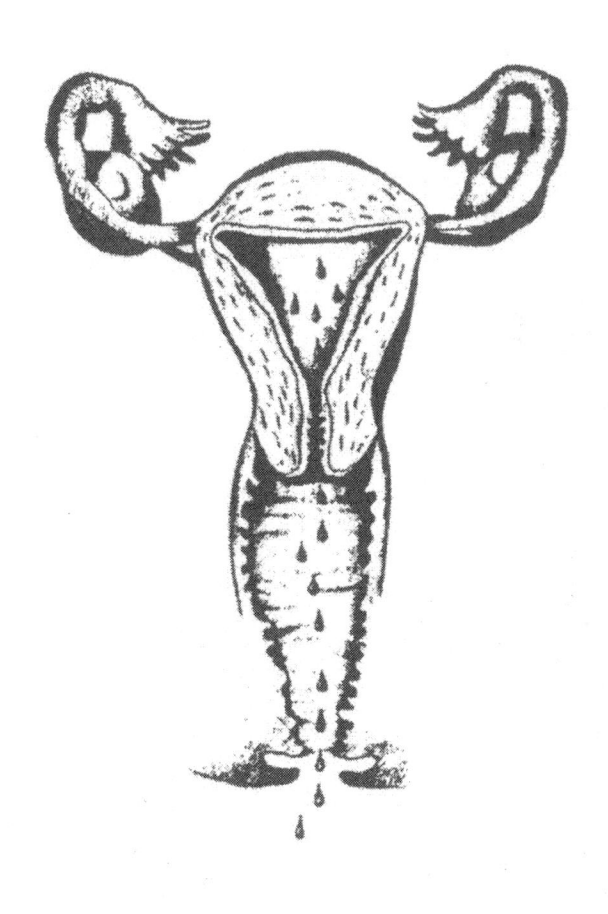

However, if a pregnancy has begun to form, there will be no shedding of the endometrial layer, nor will it be regenerated the following month —therefore there is no bleeding.

In spite of this, sometimes there can be some spotting during pregnancy, especially during the first few weeks. This is often mistaken for a "different" menstruation and is known as implantation bleeding.

This is usually small in quantity and short in duration —much shorter than the usual menstrual bleeding. However, it can be heavier and, in such cases, it is really confusing to precisely determine if it is a regular menstruation or the aforementioned event. On the other hand, although usually this only happens at the beginning, some pregnant women say that they "menstruated," or had their period, for several months of their pregnancy.

In actuality, menstruation and pregnancy are incompatible, that is, if there is menstruation, there is no pregnancy and vice versa. But, since science is at times capricious, nobody knows if some day in the future we will have to admit that those patients who have insisted that they had their period during gestation were right, while those of us who are educated in the actual scientific knowledge emphatically argued with them all along that it was not possible. Beyond this almost philosophical discussion, the arrival of menstruation certainly brings up many questions for adolescent girls.

Frequently Asked Questions

At what age does it start? How many days should it last? How often should it happen? How should you act during those days? Is it painful?

So many questions! The problem is that in the years before adolescence, there are no major changes, except for growth. However, all of a sudden, so many things happen at once that there is almost no time to react. I am going to help you find answers to these and other worries that young women usually have during this time.

The first menstruation, for example, can appear as early as age nine or be delayed until age sixteen, which depends on many factors. In any case, it is normal for it to appear any time during this wide age range.

When the first bleeding occurs before nine years of age, medical examination should always be done in order to investigate the causes. They are really simple to investigate and also to resolve. They range from a slight trauma or some infection, all the way up to other causes that are theoretically more complicated and almost always associated with disorders in the production or functioning of the hormones. The causes usually have to do with some inadequate hormonal stimulation in the organs responsible for the establishment of the menstrual cycle. These cases should always be treated by the gynecologist. In medical language, menstruation that appears before age nine is called precocious or premature menarche.

If the start of menstruation is delayed until sixteen years of age, this also should prompt a visit to the doctor, because by this age there is no physiological reason for the first menstruation not to appear. Of course some diagnoses are somewhat complicated, but if this is your situation, do not be afraid because, most times, just a simple treatment can resolve the situation.

According to multiple research investigations done on different populations in various countries, normal menstruation lasts between two and eight days, and the volume of flow varies greatly, from just a few spots every day to a copious amount of bleeding. It is good for you to know that it is as normal to scarcely bleed as it is to bleed abundantly —unless the bleeding seems excessive, in which case you might need the opinion of a gynecologist.

A gynecologist? Yes, of course. The gynecologist does not exists solely to attend to adult women. Young girls and adolescent girls can also have problems related to their reproductive systems, and the gynecologist is the right specialist to treat them. Therefore you should not have any doubts about going to see a gynecologist.

If you go to the dictionary, you will see that menstruation comes from menstrual, from the Latin *menstrualis,* which means "monthly." That is, it is a cyclical process that repeats, approximately every twenty-eight days. Of course, it does not occur this way in every woman. Some will have shorter cycles, menstruating every twenty-four days, and others longer cycles, with menstruations every thirty-two days. All these variations are normal.

In adolescent girls, menstrual cycles can be longer. It is not unusual for a month to pass without a menstruation. This should not be a cause for worry. The first two or three years after the first menstruation appears, the body is adjusting that part of its complex machinery, until it succeeds in properly establishing the menstrual cycle, and by that time, menstruation will become regular, occurring every month.

Since it is hard to know when menstruation will start, it is recommended that young women always carry sanitary napkins in their purses, to avoid being surprised and ending up with blood stains on their clothes.

Another thing you should know about menstruation is that at times it may show up as a slight discomfort in the lower part of the abdomen. However, most of the time, blood flows during the whole period without you even noticing, precisely because it is a normal process of the female organism. But occasionally, the discomfort can be painful, and the pain can become repetitive. In these cases you should visit an adolescent gynecologist so that he or she can give you the proper guidance.

What I am explaining is very important because sometimes mothers and grandmothers will tell adolescents that these pains are normal, since they suffered from them in their time, and they will not take you to see the gynecologist. It is good for you to know that not all pain is normal and, in some cases, lack of proper and timely treatment can cause a number of disorders in the sexual and reproductive health of young women: from just self-consciousness, all the way to undesirable difficulties in having children when they decide to do so. Because of this, in the case of chronic pain related to the menstrual period, even if you do not consider it intense, do not fail to seek the guidance of a specialist.

What About Hygiene?

In spite of the fact that menstruation is an absolutely normal process, it is very important to maintain adequate hygiene during this time. In fact, this is the only change that adolescent girls (adult women also, of course) should make in their habits during these days.

When there is no menstruation, rinsing the area with water is sufficient upon waking up and during bath or shower time, because if you do this too much, you could interfere with the natural barrier that protects the vagina from germs. Then those germs could penetrate it and elevate the risk of infection.

While menstrual bleeding is going on, things change, because during this time the secretions that are normally produced in this area are stronger, so rinsing should be more frequent.

Another important thing that you should never forget is that rinsing of the genital area should always be done from front to back. Remember that the anus is very near and if you are not conscious of that, the germs that normally live in that area can be dragged to the entrance of the vagina and cause vaginal infections.

Years ago, in some countries, mothers and grandmothers used to teach their daughters and granddaughters some totally mistaken lessons related to menstruation, which definitely are past history: "it is forbidden to wash your hair during menstruation," "you should not walk barefoot because you will catch cold," and other such legends. These fears are far from reality, because for as many days as the menstrual period lasts, young women can carry on with their completely normal lives without restrictions of any type, since menstruation is a normal physiological process of the female sex.

The Calendar

There is another very important thing to have in mind from this moment forward, and it is the tracking of the menstrual cycle. From the moment menstruation starts, it is a good practice to always have a calendar in your purse or to put one in a visible spot in your room in order to make a note of the day of the month that your menstruation starts and its duration.

This is a very useful practice that will serve you well, because once the cycles are established, it will help you to know the approximate date that your next menstruation will start, and in the case of some disorder or just a simple doubt, the existence of this calendar will make it easy for you and the gynecologist to interpret the problem, if you have to go see him or her.

Remember that, at first, while the complex mechanism required for the normal functioning of the menstrual cycle is adjusting, bleeding can be irregular —that is, the next menstrual period can be late or come early. When doubts about the normalization of the cycle appear, if you have not carefully kept track of the duration and frequency of your menstrual period, it will be more difficult for the gynecologist to guide you.

You already know, for example, that it is normal during this initial stage to go two months without menstruating, or to go in the opposite direction and menstruate twice in the same month. Many times this disorder fixes itself as time passes and does not even require treatment. But as the years pass, when you start to have sexual intercourse, this habit of rigorously keeping track of those days in your calendar will serve as an alert when you see that the cycle is late, which may mean that you have started a pregnancy.

I tell you this last thing because during adolescence, all precautions should be taken to avoid pregnancy. You should also know that the most important thing when you start to be sexually active is to always use contraceptive protection, especially *condoms*, which not only prevent a pregnancy, but also protect you from sexually transmitted infections, which always bring bad consequences. Later I will talk to you about them.

All that I have explained to you about menstruation is also of interest for adolescent boys because by being aware of these things they can help their girlfriends track their menstrual cycle.

EJACULATION

In the female body, ovulation should take place each month, a process which releases an ovum, an egg, ready to be fertilized. But I also told you that the presence of sperm is necessary to complete fertilization, so now I will explain to you how ejaculation is produced in boys. Ejaculation is the output of semen, with its ample content of sperm ready to fertilize the egg.

The ejaculation center is located in the lumbar region of the spinal cord —that is, in the lower part of spine— and its actions depend on a complex control mechanism of the nervous system also directed by the all-powerful brain.

The glans of the penis constitutes one of the important elements in the process of ejaculation, because it is equipped with a highly organized sensory system. It is very receptive to touch and very easily stimulated when it is touched. When sexual stimulation is initiated, the corpus cavernosum fills up with blood and, in a very short time, produces an erection in the penis. These sensations that are felt, be it because of a touch, rubbing against something, or caresses, etc., send messages to the brain through the spinal cord. When sexual excitement reaches maximum intensity, the reflexes respond with other messages that are translated into contractions in the testicles, epididymis, and vas deferens, which eject the sperm toward the urethra.

Surely you have no doubt about where the testicles are, but if you forgot exactly where it is that the epididymis and the vas deferens are running around, take a look at the illustrations again.

While this is happening, the seminal vesicle and the prostate muscle are also experiencing contractions, as well as the muscles of the pelvis, causing an expulsion through the penis of approximately 3 to 5 ml of a viscous fluid, which is the semen, along with its sperm content.

The sperm are smaller than the ovum. Each ejaculation ejects them from the body through the urethra in a quantity that varies from fifty thousand to one hundred and fifty thousand.

During the brief moments when these contractions are happening, the man experiences the most pleasurable sensations of the entire sexual intercourse, and this is what is called the male orgasm, also known in popular language as "to come," "to finish," and other such expressions.

Nocturnal Ejaculation

As I mentioned before, once your development begins, the testicles work continuously, and they do not stop producing sperm, which are stored little by little until there comes a moment when the "warehouse" is full. When this happens, the control mechanisms of the nervous system become active, unleashing an ejaculation without the help of any external sexual stimulus.

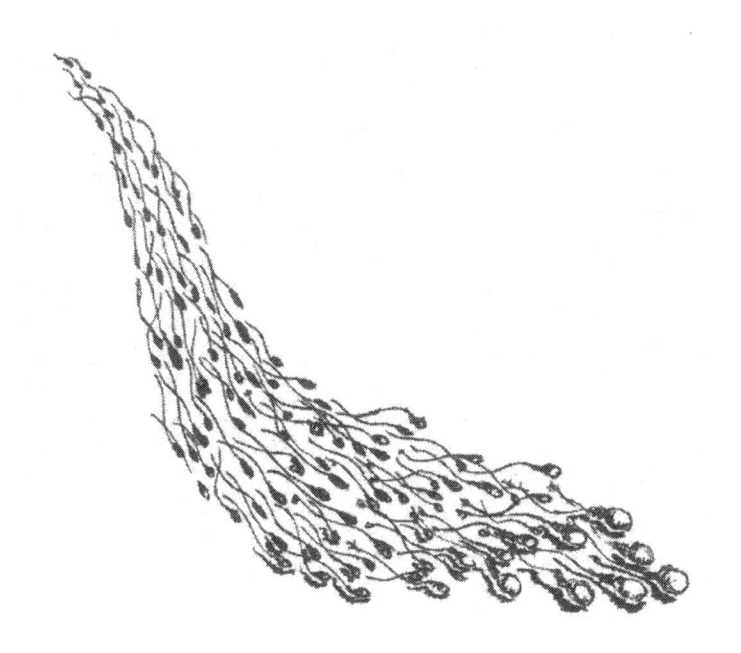

Sperm

Most of the time, this involuntary ejaculation surprises boys when they are asleep, and it is because of this that they sometimes wake up with the sheets stained by a viscous secretion, which is precisely the semen expelled during sleep.

During the emission of the semen, even without any physical stimulus at that moment, young men can wake up experiencing nice sensations of pleasure, and this is completely normal. The involuntary release of semen can happen at any time during the day, but it can be more frequent during sleep. Generally it is given the name "nocturnal."

On the other hand, even though it is truly more frequent in adolescents, it is known that it can happen to men of any age.

SEXUAL ACTIVITY DURING ADOLESCENCE

When we are small we like to think about "when I get big," and we play games about being "grown-ups." But in adolescence, many times we believe we are big —the equivalent of believing that we are adults— and at that moment, we still are not.

The difference is that when we are still children, everything is nothing more than a simple game, but in adolescence things change, because we have to look at things in a different way, and many times we think we know all that we need to know, and it really is not like that.

In these marvelous years of changes and more changes, maybe you have not even noticed that you have begun to make some decisions on your own without having to depend on your parents at all, like you did during childhood. This is something truly important in your journey toward adulthood. Now you can decide what clothes to wear, what hairdo you will have, and which movie you want to see. In fact, spontaneously, little by little —and forever— that imaginary umbilical cord, which was still connecting you to your parents, begins to break. But during this phase, as for the rest of your life, many times we are faced with difficult decisions —even the adults are— and in these cases it is most prudent to carefully think about each step before making a definite decision about a specific situation. And without doubt, you should consult your parents, even when you think that the "old folks" are already "out of fashion." When they were your age, they also lived through many experiences; therefore, there is no question that they are the best choice to guide you and to prevent you from making the wrong decision, because it is also true that in adolescence we often confuse what we should do with what we *believe* we should do. This sounds like a tongue twister, but this is the way it is.

When we were children, for example, we went everywhere in the company of our moms and dads, but the time came when we could go around on our own, and then we started hanging out with our friends from the neighborhood and from school. This was also the time of our first girlfriend and boyfriend relationships.

Until just recently, your parents knew where you were every minute and, of course, knew what you were doing, because you were always with them. But time passes, and now your parents know where you are, but they do not know what you are doing. This difference is not as simple as it seems. It signifies that, by this time, you have to have already learned what you should do and what you shouldn't do. It happens that during this time of your life, once you are an adolescent, your parents are concerned about you precisely because you are growing, and this means that you are making decisions, sometimes without consulting them.

When you were small, you were more defenseless, because you depended completely on your parents. Now you are more vulnerable, and this difference is important because it means that you have learned to cross the street, to care for your clothes, to defend yourself if someone makes fun of you, and many other things. But you never before faced the possibility, or had the capacity, to make your own decisions, which, sometimes, can even be different than the ones your mom and dad want you to make.

During these years, in addition to the biological changes that I have been analyzing, there are also other important changes taking place in your relationship with the world around you. Now is the time to decide what you should and should not do. Think about it this way: you are leaving childhood behind, and from this moment forward, life will have new challenges and new horizons, therefore, the decisions you make during this time will always be important, since they will define, in great measure, the path you choose to take.

The preparation for adult life will continue through adolescence, but our main duty should continue to be schoolwork, even though we will also be preparing for the moment when we will have sexual relations and, in the future, marry and have children.

But notice that what I said was "we will be preparing for," not that we should be initiating sexual relations, because we are still only adolescents.

Sex Without Intercourse

In the first few pages of this book I was saying that the brain was something like the orchestra director and that nothing gets done in our body that is not ordered by it. From that we could arrive at the conclusion that the brain not only has to do with the biological functions of our body, but also with absolutely all we do. That means that, each and every decision we make is also the total responsibility of the brain.

The difference —a very important one of course— between the functions of the heart, the lungs, etc., and the ones related to our thinking and analytical capacity, is that we cannot decide the volume of blood that comes into and out of the heart or how much oxygen we breath, but we can decide what we do, when we do it, and how we do it.

This capacity that human beings have to be able to decide our actions is something marvelous, because it allows us to choose between the different paths that destiny offers us. In life, we encounter many situations. Some of them are unexpected, and the capacity to decide which way we are going to act upon them will determine what the results of our actions will be.

During this time, in effect, we are preparing for adult life, and it is time to put to practice new ways to express our feelings, and to that end we should know that there are many ways to communicate, as well as give and receive affection. Kisses, hugs, and caresses produce a lot of satisfaction for young couples, without necessarily having to include sexual relations that include penis penetration. Kissing, for example, is a very common way to express feelings toward another person of the opposite sex (or of the same sex, according to sexual preference). Those first kisses in the dark, in the intimacy of mutual attraction, are a gift from nature.

When we kiss and caress the person we have chosen —and who chose us, of course— as the person with whom we want to share a closer relationship, we feel extraordinarily good.

We experience a thrill all over our body and a moment of such pleasure that we never want it to end. It is possible to feel this excitement without the need to go "all the way," like we sometimes call sexual relations with penetration.

The orgasm, which is the moment that culminates sexual relations —that instant that is the most intense and thrilling of all the various sexual contacts— can be perfectly achieved by both members of the couple when they both have a great desire to get as close as possible.

The man, as well as the woman, has the capacity to have an orgasm, and penetration of the penis into the vagina is not necessary to achieve it, although, many times young men decide the opposite with the objective of convincing their girlfriend to please them. Be very careful about pressuring your partner!

Boys usually pressure their girlfriends into sexual relations with penetration, but it also happens that in group conversations among peers, of girls as well as boys, those who have started sexual relations try to convince those who have not yet experienced them to do it. This is a pretty common characteristic of adolescence: to do what everybody else is doing. The worst thing is, we do not even think, so here is where our maturity is put to the test, as is our capacity to be able to say "no" when we have to. Will you have enough maturity to decide for yourself, or will you be lured by your pushy peer group? Maybe this is the moment when we put our personality to the test regarding our true sense of responsibility.

During the intense years of adolescence, you will, in some way, face one of these pressure situations that will put you at the crossroads of deciding to have intercourse —without really wanting to or needing to— or not to listen to your peer group. If you do not know what to do at that moment, this situation will be very difficult for you. That is why you should know that there are other options for sexual relations based on mutual caresses between the two partners and the stimulation of genital organs and other parts of the body, like the mouth (by kissing), the neck, the breasts, and many other areas (called erogenous zones), which generate pleasurable sensations and can even take you all the way to an orgasm. It is also good for you to know that an orgasm is not indispensable to feel good in a relationship, since very often, young people can feel very satisfied in their relationship even without experiencing this type of sensation, and this is very normal.

This type of sexual relation to which I refer, in which there is all the range of stimulating contact between the couple but no penis penetration, is called *petting* —in other words foreplay. *Petting* is frequently practiced by adolescents, and it is considered a very healthy —and safe— way of expressing sexuality.

It is not indispensable —and least of all an obligation— to have sexual relations with penetration so early, not to mention that it will not in the least change your adolescent condition. Having this kind of relationship will not make anyone more of a man or a woman. Always have in mind that in life trying to omit or bypass any developmental stage is never good. Enjoy the sexuality that corresponds to your age; you will be perfectly satisfied with that. Do not have any doubt about it.

Masturbation

I am sure that you have heard about masturbation. Maybe you have masturbated. It depends on how old you are as you read this, and that is why I want to talk about this issue a little bit, since sometimes this is something that nobody wants to talk about, as if those who masturbate are aliens, extraterrestrials.

When we talk about masturbation, we refer to, in essence, the auto-stimulation of the genitals —that is, sexual stimulation which we produce in ourselves, although it does not necessarily need to be auto-stimulation, since during sexual relations the couple can include mutual masturbation as part of sexual play.

This form or sexual satisfaction has been practiced through the ages, so much so that it is considered, after intercourse, the most extensively practiced sexual activity. However, for many, many years, masturbation was strongly condemned. The Catholic Church, for example, considers masturbation "an intrinsically and seriously disordered act," according to a reference from a Vatican declaration regarding sexual ethics published in 1975.

Up until the 1930s, even some doctors condemned masturbation, affirming that it caused depression, irritability, and even loss of eyesight. Fortunately, in actuality, these theories have not been confirmed. It is now clear that masturbation is not only safe but a completely normal sexual activity for both sexes and for all ages, which produces very pleasant sensations to those who practice it, allowing them to satisfy their sexual needs without having to engage in sexual relations with penetration. In spite of this, there are still some prejudices, and it is not often discussed among friends, no matter how close and open the friendship between them, and regardless of their ability to discuss other, even more delicate, subjects openly. It is even less likely to be discussed among young women, solely because of prejudice. It is also not very likely that parents will speak about this with their children —least of all with their daughters— and yet, research has shown that over 90 percent of men and more than 60 percent of women have practiced masturbation at some time in their lives and for any number of reasons.

During adolescence, a time when sexual impulses are strong, masturbation serves as an "escape valve" that can ease tension through auto-stimulation. On the other hand, if a couple has to be separated for an extended period of time, because one of them has to travel, it is preferable that both practice masturbation when they feel sexual desires, to avoid being dragged by their sexual impulses into the temptation of looking for a temporary new partner, with all the risks that entails. In this case, masturbation is a transitory solution in the absence of a partner, a way to maintain fidelity, and a way to avoid the risk of being infected with a sexually transmitted disease by participating in casual sexual relations with others.

In addition to that, masturbation is a common practice with many couples, who adopt it as an addition to their intimate relations. It can vary as auto-stimulation, simultaneous stimulation, or even mutual stimulation, when one partner masturbates the other. Any of these options can have the same pleasant results, as long as both partners approve.

Another reason why couples masturbate during the course of a relationship is when they want to avoid penetration of the penis into the vagina, be it as a method of birth control, to prevent a pregnancy they do not want, or simply because they consider this type of relationship sufficient since it offers them all they need, while prolonging the moment until they have their first sexual relation with penetration.

Even when this type of sexual contact is not approved by some, especially the family of adolescent women, it does constitute a really practical alternative for young couples who have active sexual desires and want to have a relationship beyond kissing and caressing, but who do not want to have sex with penetration.

They know that mutual masturbation offers them a lot of protection compared to penetration, which in a precocious sexual relationship often happens without the proper protections and therefore carries risks.

Masturbation is completely inoffensive: it does not hurt anyone, and with practice it is possible to experience pleasurable sensations that come without the associated risks of pregnancy or contracting a sexually transmitted disease.

So, there is no reason to be ashamed when this subject is mentioned, and it should be talked about at the appropriate time without false pretenses.

Anal Intercourse

In other cases, to avoid penetration of the penis into the vagina, or as part of the relationship, young people resort to another variety, which is anal intercourse. I have heard many adolescents say that this variety of sexual relations is the best for their age, because it is a way they can enjoy sex with penetration while renouncing vaginal penetration, which according to them should be avoided during adolescence, since in many cultures it is considered forbidden or sinful.

I can tell you, on principle, that this type of sexual relation is also normal. Not a small number of women consider it pleasurable and even reach orgasm that way, while others reject it because they find that it is uncomfortable or painful.

But you also need to know that though the entrance to the vagina is kept intact by utilizing the anal opening, if you are thinking this is not the moment to begin vaginal sexual relations, then it is not the moment to have anal relations either, because in the end, it is also a sexual relation with penetration and, as such, carries certain risks of which you should be well aware.

In anal intercourse there is no possibility of pregnancy because there is absolutely no direct communication with the internal genitals, but there are health risks. Some microorganisms inhabit the rectum which do not pose any problem in that zone, since this is their "home," (that is, they normally live there), but if transported to the vagina or the entrance of the urethra, these same microorganisms can cause serious infections. For this reason and in order to avoid these complications, you should never put the penis in contact with the vulva after anal intercourse.

This type of sexual relation has another risk, because the rectum is a highly vascular area, which means it has many blood vessels, and AIDS can be transmitted by blood If one of the partners is infected with this virus when having anal intercourse, the virus can very easily penetrate through these blood vessels, causing a contamination. Because of this, women carry a higher risk of contamination than men, since, regardless of how delicate the penetration, the rectal area is more easily susceptible to trauma, than the skin of the penis.

This is the reason that male homosexual couples have an elevated risk of AIDS contamination, unless they absolutely always use condoms for protection. Because of this, anal intercourse should always —pay close attention, a-l-w-a-y-s— be done with protection in order to avoid contact with semen which could be contaminated.

When to Begin Having Intercourse?

Like you have probably noticed through all that I have told you, intercourse is not the only way to feel pleasure in sexual life, besides the fact that it carries certain risks when it is done without the minimal condition required for this type of very significant union.

This is not a simple whim or an "old people's thing." Do not look at this as advice from an adult, since to you an adult represents someone who is probably "old fashioned." It is just that we must consider intercourse as the peak of the union of a couple, and it must be mediated by deep feelings of love between the two. Like everything in life, one has to be prepared for this, because there is nothing quite like the pleasant memory or our first sexual experience.

Then, surely, the question comes to mind: at what age should one start? Well, the answer is not a precise age, because sexual activity is not regulated by the calendar, like a movie which is restricted according to a specific age or a driver's license, which you must be a certain age to obtain. Nobody has ever established a minimum age that is considered the appropriate moment to initiate sexual intercourse with penetration.

However, in the last decades it has been proven that adolescents initiate sexual activity at a very young age, and this practice, as you already know, has its risks, because what usually happens is that they do not take proper precautionary measures.

Without a doubt, a relationship that includes sexual intercourse produces a lot of pleasure for a couple, but when there is no existing close and intimate relationship between the two people involved, when there is no love and not enough maturity, one should not advance to intercourse, since a moment of pleasure could turn into a real tragedy for any of you, leaving scars that, although it may be hard for you to believe, will be difficult to erase.

In various research studies, it has been proven that many adolescent girls have their first sexual intercourse out of curiosity, excitement, or simply because they are pressured by their boyfriend or their friends, like I told you a while ago. But I will insist time and time again that the only truly valid reason for giving yourself to another is love.

If you become close with someone and decide to have intercourse only because you have sexual desires, because you want to be "like everybody else," because of a physical attraction, or worse still, to realize some financial benefit in exchange for it, you will be making a grave mistake. When sex becomes the result of any of these premises that I have just mentioned, it will only lead to failure and deception, and in the end, an empty feeling that will inevitably invade you.

Under no circumstances should sexual relations turn into a simple mechanical act, because this really should be a beautiful moment of surrender to the person we love. This idea is valid for both young women and young men, although sometimes the initial moment of sexual relations is overvalued for young women, while it is minimized for young men, inciting them, in many cases, to start as soon as possible. This is a real mistake, and it demonstrates a very wrong way to look at things. It is incorrect to assume that when speaking about the proper moment to begin sexual relations there is no real difference between boys and girls of the same age. If we consider that girls at a certain age have sufficient maturity to begin sexual relations, then supposedly boys will be prepared at the same age. However, this assumes that the mental development of adolescents of both sexes is the same, when in fact quite the opposite is true: boys are still playing in the park when girls of the same age are already showing an interest in boys as boyfriends. That is the reason why, very often during this time of adolescence, girls may be attracted to boys who are older than them and sometimes even reject those who are their own age, since they consider them too immature.

Sex is with us from birth, but the way we express it is up to us and should always be mediated by feelings of love. It is true that when we are adolescents, sometimes we pay more attention to what our friends say or to what the neighborhood kids say than to our parents, but you must keep in mind that adults have a wider view of life —not because we are more intelligent, but because we have lived more... and we have already tripped and maybe even gotten hurt.

If you stop a moment to reflect, and you think that the moment has really not yet arrived, if you believe that you should wait until you feel love before you arrive at this significant union, then do not give in to pressure —and you will have made the correct decision. Do not let anyone decide for you. This will help you to be more confident in life.

The first sexual relation is a very important act in each of our lives. It is a day that is never forgotten, precisely because it was the first day you had this kind of profound and pleasant union. If you do not experience this at the right moment and with all the right conditions, this memory will never be a pleasant one, and sooner or later, you will regret having been in such a hurry.

PREGNANCY

One of the negative consequences of irresponsible sexual intercourse is an unexpected pregnancy, because adolescence is not the appropriate moment to have a child. By any means —and there are many— you should avoid gestation while you are so young, because it can only bring problems.

Pregnancy during adolescence has many risks, since from a biological point of view, during this time of life the adequate biological preparation does not exist for this complex process, much less the psychological preparation.

For Girls

If we consider this only from a strictly biological point of view, young women can get pregnant during adolescence, because once the ovulation cycle starts, a pregnancy is possible. Any adolescent woman can know which month of what year she will begin her ovulation cycle, so she should be careful.

Carlos Ortiz Lee

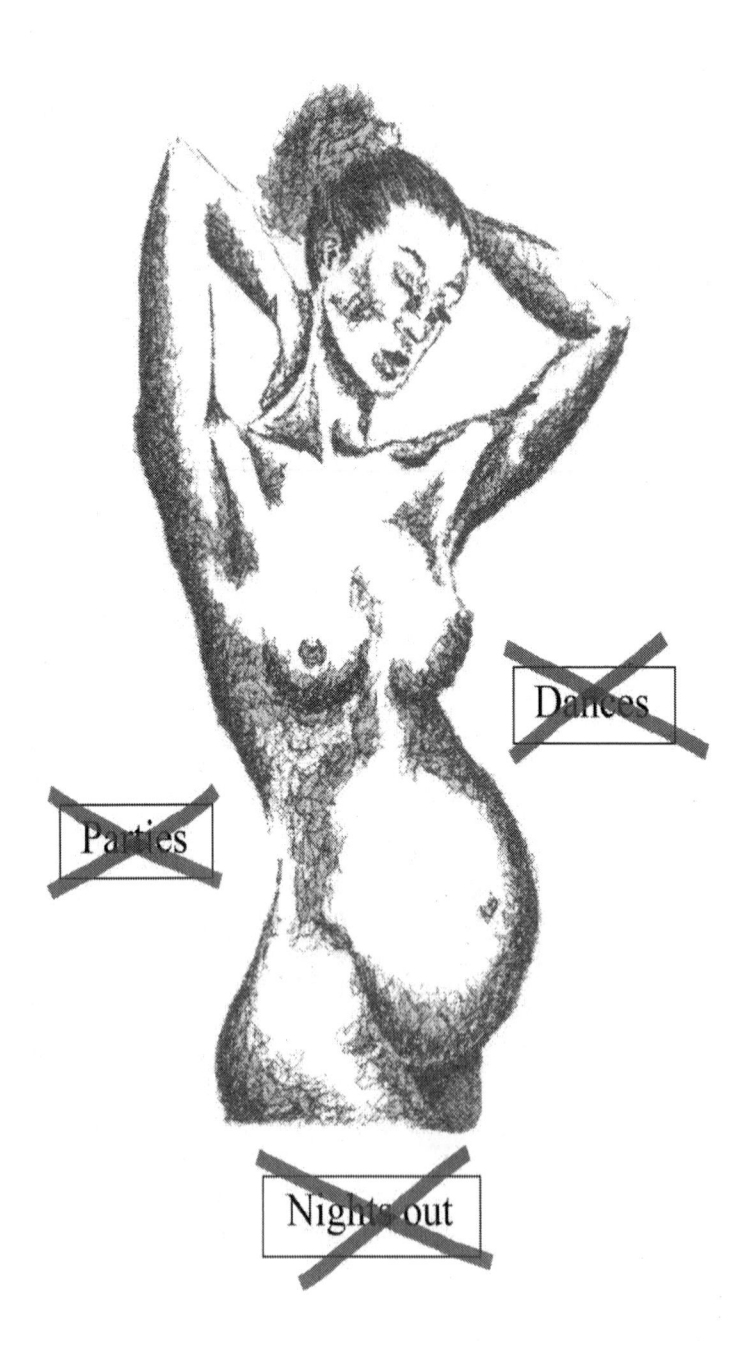

Just because you are already menstruating does not mean anything, because the body, and specifically the reproductive system, are still not mature enough for that, and you would only expose yourself to some very serious health risks, since adolescent girls who are pregnant have a higher probability of developing complications than adult women. Remember that adolescence is a period of deep biological transformation, which is the reason why during this time there is a greater possibility of developing diseases like anemia, pregnancy-related high blood pressure, and other afflictions that threaten the prognosis of the pregnancy.

Risks exist also at the moment of delivery because you may need to have a caesarean section, which has a higher risk of complications than a vaginal delivery. But even if you are able to have a vaginal delivery, you are still exposed to some risks, like tearing of the neck of the uterus, the vagina, and the perineum. It is true that with the number of doctors we have now who specialize in these conditions, these risks have minimized, but you will always face a higher probability of any type of complication than adult women face.

On the other hand, these risks are not only true for you, but your child will also have greater possibility of presenting problems, especially the risk of being born below normal weight, be it due to a premature delivery or, even if the child is born full-term, due to the effects of deficient intrauterine nutrition caused by an immature reproductive system. For any of these reasons, the child could even die shortly after birth. I do not like to exaggerate, but it has been proven that major complications exists in children of adolescent mothers, and the younger they are, the worse the risks.

Sometimes we only focus on the physical complications that adolescent mothers, as well as the newborns can have, and we forget that from a social point of view, pregnancy at this age can also have important implications. Close your eyes and give free rein to your imagination: imagine that you are pregnant and that you are sitting in the classroom at your school.

What would be happening with you? If you are experiencing the discomfort that is frequently present during the first few months of pregnancy, you would have to miss class, and if your doctor recommends a prolonged rest like sometimes happens, you could even miss your current school year.

The moment will come when you can no longer participate in sports, which is so important to your development, and if the pregnancy is during exam time, it will be difficult to find the time to get a passing grade while your adolescence is being spent on diaper changing and sleepless nights. You will have to say good-bye to parties, to dances, and to going out at night with your friends. Finally, this beautiful time of life, when we can have so much fun, will be over for you, so you can dedicate your life to motherhood, which is a great responsibility when you take it seriously.

In addition, according to the circumstances, you will also have to figure out if you can continue your education while someone other than you assumes financial responsibility for your child, or if you definitely have to put your education aside and start working at whatever job you can find that will adjust to your lack of education in order to support this little creature that arrived in your life before it was time, because you will probably not be able to study and work at the same time, like many young people do. If you think about it carefully, it is better to leave pregnancy for later.

As a last resort, if you could not avoid it, you could attempt to terminate the pregnancy, but this choice through any of the methods that exist to realize it, also has risks and complications that can leave in its wake the inability to have children in the future —and can even lead to death, even if this seems like an exaggeration. Besides, there are some places where abortion is prohibited, and this could be a problem if you want to terminate the pregnancy.

Various methods exist toward this end, some more aggressive than others. This depends, among other things, on which instruments are utilized to do it and how far along the pregnancy is. Of all these methods, one that is often utilized in many countries is suction aspiration for early pregnancy. With this method, the entrance to the vagina, its walls, and the external orifice of the uterine neck are carefully cleansed to avoid infections related to the use of the instruments, and all the material corresponding to the early pregnancy is suctioned or aspirated.

In the very early stage of a pregnancy, it is sufficient to aspirate for some three minutes in order to totally extract the pregnancy, but later in pregnancy anesthesia is required, and many times this method must be completed by using a hook-shaped knife called a curette to terminate the pregnancy.

There are risks with both methods, because they are maneuvers that the specialist is doing inside the uterus, in a place where he or she cannot directly see what he or she is doing.

The suction curette and curette are long thin instruments that are introduced deep into the uterus, and there they begin their work: the suction aspires, and the curette scrapes, progressively extracting all the material that makes up that recently initiated pregnancy. Here is precisely where the danger starts, because either the suction or the scrapping may not completely remove all the material, leaving some material called "residual" inside the uterus, which can provoke an infection and the need to perform another scrapping which will multiply the risks. Or the opposite may happen: excessive scrapping can damage the interior walls of the uterus.

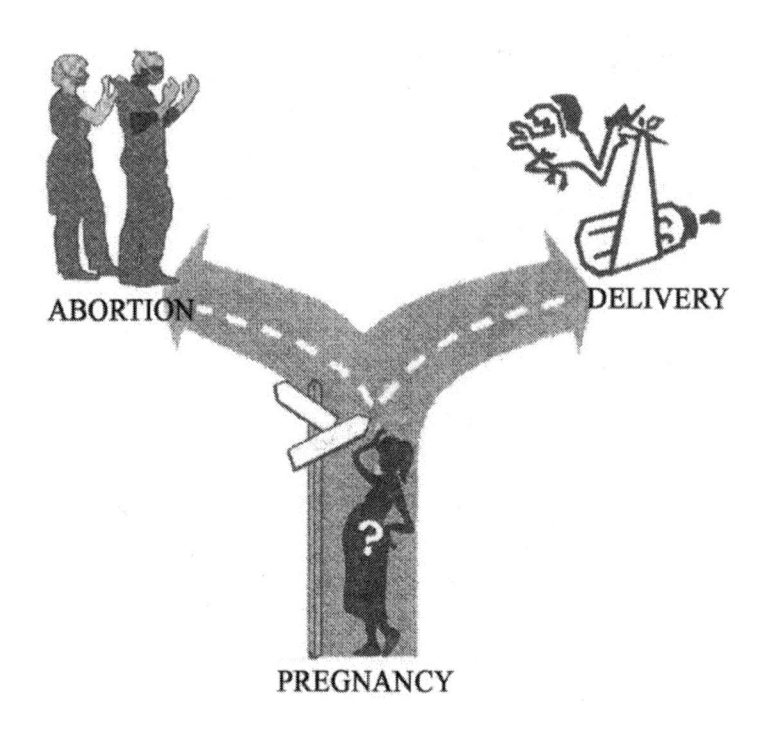

ABORTION

DELIVERY

PREGNANCY

This damage is sometimes difficult to resolve in the long run and reduces the possibility of pregnancy in the future.

There is also the possibility of accidental perforation of the uterus with one of these instruments, and this accident may be more or less serious. Sometimes it is only a simple perforation, which is treated only with observation and some measures to avoid an infection. It would usually show up in the first few days following this unpleasant event. In other cases, the perforation is more complex, be it because there are multiple perforations, because of where it is, or due to uncontrolled bleeding. In many of these patients, emergency surgery is required to resolve the problem, which can even include having to perform a hysterectomy —that is, the removal of the uterus— and at this point, the patient loses any possibility of having children in the future.

Other times, everything ends up apparently well, without any residual or perforation of the uterus, and in spite of that, an infection develops. On the other hand, in the case of curettage, the use of the anesthesia required for this procedure also carries risk for adolescent girls.

These are some examples —only some— of the multiple complications that can be produced as a consequence of a termination of pregnancy, which unfortunately some women use as an alternate method of birth control without being conscious of the risk they are taking.

Other methods of pregnancy interruption exist, but all have a degree of generally inherent complications. The other important issue is that the earlier the interruption, the lower the possibility of complications, at least theoretically. Besides, for the more advanced pregnancies, some of these methods cannot be used, and the ones that are used really complicate everything much more, from the actual procedure to the psychological aftermath. When the pregnancy develops and the fetus progresses in size, the extraction becomes more complicated, and the psychological impact is greater. With a longer pregnancy, the patient feels that she has lived a long time with the pregnancy —that is, she has had time to internalize the idea that a baby has been growing in her belly, and when she finally decides to terminate the pregnancy, the trauma tends to be major.

Up to here I have made comments on some of the important issues about the biological complications of pregnancy interruption. But I would like to talk a little more about this abortion matter, since interrupting a pregnancy is much more than lying down on a gynecological table to let some doctor solve your problem.

Interrupting the development of a pregnancy means, above all else, stopping the course of a life that has already begun to take shape. This concept, regrettably, is seldom given the importance it deserves. Pregnancy, in every case, should be the result of a well thought-out decision by the couple and in no way the result of an irresponsible sexual relationship. Be aware that "this thing" that is growing there is a child, not a toy. Think that this child who has started to gestate did not ask for this, and without it having been responsible for it, we are forcing it not to be born. Does it not make more sense to avoid this complicated situation altogether?

In my personal and professional life I have known women who have, for the rest of their lives, regretted that they were not responsible when they started to have sexual relations, because the years have passed, and they have had to face the bitter surprise of not being able to have children, as a result of complications caused by a termination of a pregnancy.

On the other hand, as you probably know, there are some countries that absolutely prohibit the practice of legal abortion and others where it depends on special or local regulations of a specific province or state.

Apart from all that, the ideal situation would be that, any place in the world, we should be conscious about the importance of avoiding unwanted pregnancies.

In those places that have established regulations about abortion, more care should well be taken, since in those places, unexpected pregnancies that the patients decide to terminate end up in the always dangerous path of an illegal abortion. It would not be a gross exaggeration to say that an illegal abortion is one of the easiest and surest ways to severe health complications, including death. Believe me that this is the way it is, because in this case, the statistics speak for themselves.

When people are desperate to have an abortion, sometimes they are done in inappropriate places, by people who do not have the professional capability to realize this medical procedure, and sometimes this result in the improper use of aseptic and antiseptic methods. Also, these clandestine places are frequently not equipped with the necessary means to handle the immediate complications of the procedure, and if a patient requires emergency surgery, it is not at all simple to resolve the problem.

It would be better for you to avoid sexual intercourse until the required conditions exist for this type of union, but once you decide to initiate it, you and your partner together should have a conversation to immediately choose an appropriate method of preventing a pregnancy. Notice that I am saying "together," because sometimes adolescents think that avoiding pregnancy is just the girl's problem, and this constitutes a big mistake. In the same way that intercourse takes the two of you, both of you have the same level of responsibility when it is time to avoid a pregnancy.

If your partner is not capable of understanding that, he or she is decidedly not the person with whom you should initiate sexual relations.

Another important thing is that this conversation should happen at the very moment when you start considering if you are going to have sexual intercourse. Under no circumstances should you "leave it for later," because statistics show that pregnancy usually shows up, in more than 50 percent of cases, in the first six months after initiating sexual relations. Remember that you only need to have sex once to produce a pregnancy.

With the advice of your parents and teachers, the explanations that I have offered so far, plus the guidelines about contraceptives that you will read in the upcoming pages, there is no reason for you to be included in that long list of statistics about precocious pregnancies that I just mentioned, which bring such unpleasant memories to those who have lived through such a bitter experience.

For Boys

Although you do not run the risk of becoming pregnant by having unprotected sex and therefore are not exposed to the biological implications or the associated complications that an adolescent pregnancy brings, this is an aside for the boys about the subject of pregnancy. If you read carefully in the first part of this chapter when I spoke to the girls, you would have noticed that when an adolescent girl becomes pregnant, she is risking even her very life. Think about it —this young woman could be your fiancé or your sister.

What right do you have to put someone else's life at risk? How would you feel if she were to encounter some of the complications that can show up during pregnancy? Probably sad and sorry, but, worse, you would always carry the burden of that unpleasant memory of something that both of you could have avoided.

In order for these things not to happen, you should act with maturity, and when you finally decide to initiate sexual relations, then you should not have intercourse without adequate contraceptive protection. Be aware that I insist again and again about the same thing because it is very important that you act responsibly when the time comes to decide about this. In this way, your girlfriend will feel more secure, and your relationship with her will be closer, because she will know that you care for her.

Even before you start having sex with intercourse, you should always be very careful, because remember that sometimes a pregnancy can be produced even without penis penetration into the vagina. This is called a "virginal pregnancy," and it is more common than you imagine.

How can this be possible? It is very simple. Sometimes, with the best of intentions, adolescent couples limit themselves to a passionate exchange of kisses and caresses without penis penetration, but this contact sometimes ends in ejaculations, and although it is not inside the vagina, it is no less risky, so be very careful with that! If during the moment of ejaculation, the semen ends up on the external part of the vagina, near its entrance, even on the thighs, it is not at all unusual that a pregnancy be produced, because the sperm has a lot of mobility, like I already explained. When a young man reaches orgasm, the moment that produces the expulsion of semen, if the pertinent precautions have not been taken, the sperm can, as unbelievable as it seems, go up and end up fertilizing the ovum, and a pregnancy can show up in this way. Be aware of this possibility, which is not infrequent, and avoid it.

For Both

According the calculations of the World Health Organization (WHO), some one hundred million pregnancies are created daily. Of these, one in every two hundred is unplanned, and one in every four hundred is not wanted. Adolescent pregnancies are, of course, included in these numbers, and there are a lot.

In adult couples, an unplanned pregnancy sometimes happens, but although it is unplanned, it is wanted since the required conditions exist to face this beautiful moment of life that pregnancy is. But in adolescence, what usually happens is that the pregnancy is not planned, let alone wanted, during this time of life.

Statistics, with their often alarming numbers, also inform us that some hundred abortion-related deaths are recorded worldwide on a daily basis, and another hundred are recorded daily for causes related to pregnancy.

There are only two ways to avoid an unplanned pregnancy: not having sexual relations with intercourse and, once initiated, never, under any circumstance, failing to use some method of contraception.

I am going to make some comments about this interesting subject in the following pages.

CONTRACEPTIVE METHODS

There are different methods used to prevent a pregnancy. Most of them are designed for women, but that does not mean that boys do not have the responsibility to look for adequate contraceptive protection: absolutely the contrary. I already told you that pregnancy is a couple's problem, because so far I have not found any women who have become pregnant without male participation.

There are hormonal contraceptives that are administered in tablet form, through injections, and also in the form of subdermal implants, which are placed superficially under the skin. In the last few years, patches have also become popular; these deliver a slow and consistent release of hormones that prevent fertilization. But patches are still too new to be recommended for adolescents, because they have been surrounded by some contradictions. That is why I only mention them, so that you are aware that they exist, but I am not going to refer to this option again.

In all cases, hormonal contraceptives are made up of different doses, which have the common objective of inhibiting ovulation and, in that way, preventing pregnancy.

There are tablets containing varying concentrations of hormones, but the one most used in recent years for adolescents is called "the combined pill," which for doctors call in different ways, but we better not speak in such terms in order not to tangle this up, since the classification of the different types of hormonal contraceptives is a little complicated, so we better keep talking about the parts that interest you.

Packages can have from twenty-one to twenty-eight tables. If they have twenty-one pills, they should be started from the fifth day of menstruation, taking seven days off before starting the next package; while the ones that have twenty-eight tablets should be taken from the first day of menstruation, without taking a break between packages. They are taken continuously every day for as long as one wants to continue using this method of contraception, which is very effective. With any of these varieties, the pills should be ingested at approximately the same time every day in order to be safe.

One of the disadvantages of this pill method is that it must be accompanied by a good memory, in a way that those who decide to use them must have a serious sense of responsibility. When one or more pill is forgotten, bleeding can appear, but the most worrisome is the risk of pregnancy.

There are a few issues that you should take into account if you decide to use one of the many contraceptive pills when you initiate sexual relations with intercourse:

- If you forget to take the pill, you should take one as soon as you realize that you forgot then continue to take the next one at the usual time, even if this means that you take two tablets on the same day.
- If you forget to take more than one pill, take one as soon as you realize it, suspend sexual intercourse, and visit your gynecologist immediately for guidance.

Also, during the first three months after you start using oral contraceptives, some unpleasant effects may appear which doctors call "side effects." These can be the appearance of slight bleeding or spotting between one menstruation and the next, nausea, dizziness, slight headaches, and tenderness in the breasts. Generally, these symptoms disappear in short order, so these symptoms should not be a reason for interrupting this method.

Contraceptive injections, for their part, have the same effects as the pills, and they can be administered once a month every two months or every three months, depending on the hormonal concentration they contain. They have the advantage of reducing the risk of forgetting, but they sometimes can present menstrual disorders after they are administered. When these occur, sometimes they disappear spontaneously in a short time, just as they do with pill use. The really important thing in these cases is that they do not pose any type of health risk, and with a little patience, these side effects disappear after the first few cycles.

As you may know, there are many people in the world who believe that they know a little about everything, and frequently you will run into a few that are not very partial to hormonal contraceptive methods. They have the wrong ideas about the use of contraceptive pills and injections, and they will tell you that using hormones is bad, that if you take them for too long you may not be able to have children, and a series of false comments about this contraceptive method. But, in reality, all the research that has been done on hormonal contraceptives (and there really has been a lot of it) disproves these beliefs.

The use of these pills not only prevents pregnancy with a very high percentage of effectiveness, but it also helps to regulate menstrual disorders, which are relatively common in adolescence, in addition to having other positive effects on general health. It may seem contradictory to you that in the previous paragraphs I told you that sometimes they cause bleeding, and now I am telling you that it serves to fix menstrual disorders. There is no contradiction in this, because the bit about those initial disorders is just at the beginning of your period, let's say the adjustment period, but sooner or later, it is really a very sure way to control menstrual cycle disorders.

In spite of that, there is a small group of adolescent girls that should not use hormonal contraception, because this method has some contraindications. For this reason, when you think about initiating any hormonal method, you should have some basic guidance like the counseling services on reproductive health, which most countries offer. Therefore you have the adequate information about the best method to choose.

On the other hand, many of the young women who use the oral contraceptive method after a while decide to stop using it for a few months in order to give their body a break from hormones. In this case, it is important for you to understand that exactly the opposite is true: while on the pill, the ovaries are being allowed to "rest," since they are not ovulating until the method is discontinued.

Another very important thing in relation to the pills is that once you start a package you should not, under any circumstance, stop taking them until the package is completely finished, because if you stop before all the pills in the package have been used, you will have problems with your menstrual cycle, like unexpected bleeding that is generally heavy. When for some reason you think you should stop ingesting the pills, your first step is a visit to the gynecologist, who can tell you what actions to take.

Intrauterine devices (IUD), like the name indicates, are placed inside the uterus. Multiple types exist, different forms and sizes, which are very effective contraceptives. For many years IUDs were not recommended for adolescents, especially because of the risk of pelvic inflammatory disease. However, new investigations are turning off that concept, because research did not find this kind of risk in adolescents. So, when doctors decide to place IUDs in adolescents, they just have to follow a similar protocol that they use for adult patients.

First of all, we have to be sure that the patient has no vaginal infection. If a vaginal infection exists at the time that the IUD is inserted, as easy and carefully done as the placement may be, the germs will be dragged toward the interior of the uterine cavity by the device on its way through the vagina and the cervical canal. In this manner, the young woman is exposed to an infection of the internal genitals. This can produce a pelvic inflammation, which can cause alterations in the anatomy of the fallopian tubes, increasing the risk of ectopic pregnancy (pregnancy that occurs outside the uterus) and infertility.

There is also a method called *periodic abstinence*, which can be used when one does not wish to utilize, or cannot utilize, other methods of contraception. Periodic abstinence is abstaining from intercourse during the fertile days of the cycle —that is, during the time that ovulation is taking place. Remember that ovulation happens only once during each cycle, and fertilization can only happen during those days. For some couples, because of some illness that prevents the use of hormonal contraceptives or intrauterine devices, periodic abstinence is sometimes the only option.

I am not going to describe it in detail because I do not recommend it for adolescents either. If adolescents use this method, they would have a high risk of becoming pregnant, since they often experience early or late menstruations due to the combination of having some cycles with, and others without ovulation, and also because in order for this method to be effective, it is necessary to have exact knowledge of the moment of ovulation, which is very difficult at your age.

Barrier methods for males and females, for their part, include preservatives (most commonly called condoms), the diaphragm, and spermicidal creams.

Of these, the male preservative, or condom, is the most widely used by couples of all ages, in all parts of the world, and at the same time, the most useful, because it serves the dual function of preventing pregnancy and protecting both people against sexually transmitted diseases. Most importantly, it has no contraindications, so that any couple can use this method.

Something very important for you to know is the correct way to use a condom, which is very simple but, if not adequately done, can fail.

In the first place, you must check to make sure it is not punctured. They rarely are, but it can happen. Then proceed with the placement, which should always be done while the penis is erect, being careful not to damage the condom with your nails. It should be in place before the first penetration, in order to meet its double objective, and not removed until after ejaculation, always being careful that it is removed before the erection goes down, in order to avoid contact between the semen and the vagina.

Remember what I told you about the extraordinary mobility of sperm: if you are not careful, it will be difficult to avoid a pregnancy.

The placement of the condom can be done by the young man and also by the young woman, incorporating it in foreplay before penetration.

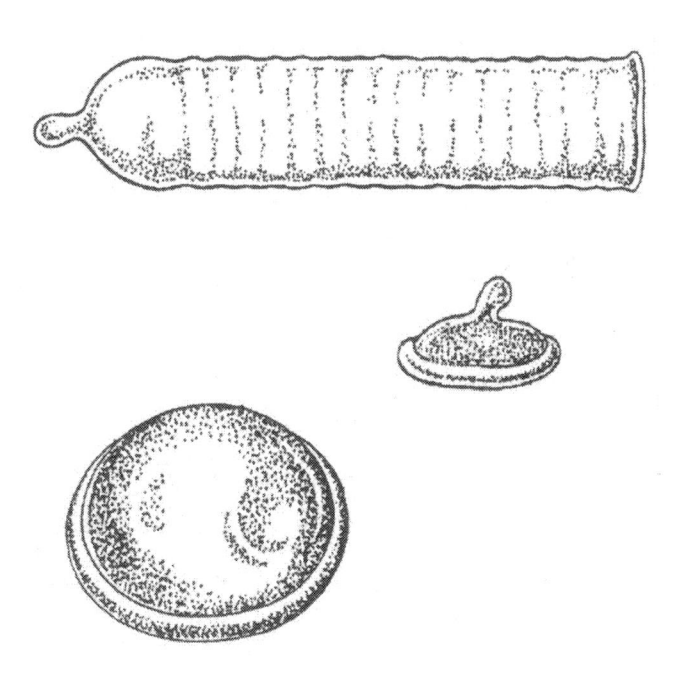

Some barrier methods

When we become accustomed to using it, we will be convinced of its utility and also understand the lies we have heard about the decrease in sensitivity of the penis, which reportedly, is experienced by condom users.

The female preservative, or diaphragm, for its part, is also effective, but its distribution is actually more limited, and it is not as easily available as the male condom. Its objective is the same, but we have to wait for greater production and greater worldwide distribution in order to hope for a more generalized use of this variety. The diaphragm is an impermeable rubber dome, which when properly placed, blocks the entrance to the cervical canal, preventing the ascent of the sperm through it. There are different forms and sizes of diaphragms, because they have to fit well in order to fulfill their function.

In order for girls to use this method (called "barrier" precisely because it serves as a barrier to impede the sperm from advancing), they must first visit the doctor, who will need to do a gynecological examination that precisely measures what size diaphragm should be used.

During that visit, the specialist will explain the details related to the way the diaphragm should be placed, when you should place it, as well as how long you should wait before you remove it, which should never be less than six hours after finishing the last intercourse or penetration. Once removed, it should be washed with soap and warm water and carefully dried before putting it away.

As you can see, it is a method that involves a series of actions before and after that must really be taken into account in order for it to be effective. It is not the most advisable method for adolescents, who sometimes arrive at the moment of intercourse before having any time to prepare even the most minimal and indispensable conditions for using a diaphragm. However, if you decide to use it, I advise using it along with a spermicide, in order to increase its effectiveness.

Spermicides are chemical agents that inactivate and kill sperm; they are available in the form of creams, jellies, and other varieties. They should not be used alone as a birth control method, because they are not as efficient, but if combined with other methods, like a condom or a diaphragm, then their effectiveness is increased.

The use of spermicidal substances, like other contraceptive methods, has its rules with which one should comply in order not to lose their effective protection.

In this sense, the most important is to follow the instructions about proper use, which vary according to each type of spermicide. This method has no contraindications, although in some cases there could be irritation due to an allergic reaction to the product.

Another method is *coitus interruptus* or the "pull-out" method, which consists of removing the penis from the vagina moments before ejaculation, in order to avoid depositing the semen in the vagina. This is not recommended for any couple, because it interrupts the moment of maximum enjoyment. Besides, many times, the penis is not removed at the exact moment, and the sperm can ascend with pregnancy as the consequence. Remember that before ejaculation a secretion is released that may contain a small amount of sperm, enough to produce a pregnancy.

This method is sometimes used as an emergency when the couple is not using any contraceptive protection and decides to have unplanned intercourse. It is necessary to avoid ending up in a situation like this. Recklessness is not a good companion.

If you are involved in a sexual relationship, and you go on vacation with your partner, you should not forget your pills or condoms, just in the same way that we do not leave behind our toothbrush or the clothes we are going to wear. We should get in the habit of including condoms in the personal things that travel with us everywhere. If they are handy, like our ID card or the keys to the house, it would be difficult for an unplanned intercourse to surprise us without this valuable protection in our pocket.

Lastly, I will mention the emergency contraception that is used when a couple has had sexual relations without adequate protection, or when the protection has failed. For example, when a condom has been improperly used, be it because it was torn or because it slipped off, when the pill was forgotten or not ingested regularly, or in any case, such as sexual violation, when we suspect that the possibility of a pregnancy exists.

Emergency contraception should be used only when faced with one of these situations, because it is not the ideal contraceptive protection.

In order to use emergency contraception, you should be aware of the possibility of using specific pills or the immediate insertion of an intrauterine device. The quicker you can implement these methods, the better your potential for success.

Levonorgestrel is the name of the medication utilized in the majority of countries where this emergency contraceptive method is used, with a dose especially designed for that use. It should be taken as soon as possible after the unprotected intercourse happens, repeating a second and equal dose twelve hours after the first. In countries where this type of medication does not exist, the same results can be achieved with the ingestion of any of the pills called "combined," which are a combination of estrogen and progesterone in their composition. In these cases, four pills should be taken together, repeating the same dose in twelve hours.

If for some reason you are considering the use of some intrauterine device, this is another variation of an emergency method that can be useful in a high percentage of cases when it is inserted in the first few days after the unprotected intercourse happens.

According to several researches, you should know that both methods have similar rates of success in emergency contraception.

The high success of these emergency methods has been confirmed, but diverse studies have revealed that the sooner after the unprotected sex they are applied, the better the possibility of preventing a pregnancy, so their true success depends upon not wasting any time before applying them. In the case of the pills, in general the ideal is that they be ingested in the first seventy-two hours after intercourse without protection; to be effective, IUD insertion should be done before five days have passed after unprotected sex.

In some countries, the distribution of these emergency pills does not require a doctor's visit, and this makes things easier, because you can save time when you need to use them.

In any case, you should not trust your luck with these last-minute methods, because they do not always work, but it is good for you to know that they exist, just in case you need them some day.

Of all these contraceptive methods, the most recommended for you are the pills and the condoms, and you really should use both, because together they increase protection: the pills prevent pregnancy even if for some reason the condom fails, and the condom offers protection from being infected by a sexually transmitted disease, which cannot be avoided using the pills alone.

After all the comments that I have made to you about contraceptives, the only thing about which I need to remind you is that, without a doubt, you will receive the best guidance about contraception at the doctor's office, and for that you do not have to wait until the moment you become sexually active, since by that time it may be too late. You should make your appointment at your earliest convenience so that you start becoming familiar with your doctor's guidance and gain some knowledge about contraceptives, a subject that will never again be foreign to you.

SEXUALLY TRANSMITTED DISEASES

Many microorganisms are capable of causing infections that are transmitted through sexual relations. Included among these are viruses, bacteria, funguses, protozoa, and even arachnids, which are very capable of easily infecting anyone.

The most well know of these is probably AIDS, which is also known as the HIV infection. It is well known due to a worldwide information campaign that exists precisely because it is considered one of the most dangerous and incurable disease in the world.

It is sad, really very sad, to know that in recent years, statistics show an ever-increasing number of adolescents who are infected because they became sexually active without taking into account adequate protective measures.

In the propaganda realized to prevent this disease, it is said that "AIDS does not have a face." However, I have a different opinion, because I believe it does have a face —and not just one, but many faces— all ugly. AIDS has the face of inexperience, of lack of knowledge, of excessive trust, and, worst, of irresponsibility.

It is known that anyone can be a carrier of this affliction, so the only way to protect ourselves is to always use a condom. According to experts in the field, the length of time that a person can live without presenting any kind of symptoms varies tremendously and can extend to many years. In all that time, that individual feels fine, like you and me. However, with each unprotected sexual act that they have, they will involuntarily infect their partner. Since we do not know who is carrying this virus, the condom —again with the condom— is our best ally.

But AIDS is not the only danger for those who do not use protection, because there is also condyloma, syphilis, gonorrhea, genital herpes, and a few others. Condyloma, also known as genital warts, are very contagious lesions that can be recognized because they are small warts, single or multiple, that appear most often on the vulva, on the walls of the vagina, on the neck of the uterus, and around the anus, while on a man, they basically show up on the penis. Treatment depends on where lesions are and how many there are.

Teenagers: growing up and sexuality

Sexual intercourse without protection

⬇
⬇

Sexually Transmitted Disease

⬇
⬇

- Inflammatory complication
- Sterility
- Blindness
- Cancer
- Mental disorders
- Death

On occasion these lesions cannot be seen with the naked eye, like the ones that appear on the walls of the vagina or the neck of the uterus, which makes diagnosis difficult. An unpredictable amount of time can pass from initial infection until they actually show up, which increases risk, since a woman can continue to have sexual intercourse and transmit the infection to each one of her partners.

With syphilis, which is caused by a bacterial contamination called Treponema pallidum, first we see a lesion called a chancre in the same place where the infection started, which spontaneously disappears without any treatment. This makes it easy to forget about it, thinking that it healed itself, when the reality is that after the lesion heals, the disease continues its course in silence without any symptoms, progressively affecting the entire body. From that moment on, those infected are exposed to severe cardiovascular and neurological disorders, which can even cause death. In the case of women, if they have a child during this time when they are not experiencing symptoms, the child will be born already infected by the mother.

Gonorrhea is another sexually transmitted infection, which is most easily detected in males because it shows up as a thick secretion through the penis, while in women it is not discovered during the initial period of the infection, since at the beginning, no secretion is produced. However, later on it can produce a severe pelvic inflammation that many times ends up being a chronic disease that can cause a periodically painful condition, affecting even the liver. It can also lead, like I already mentioned, to a dangerous ectopic pregnancy or infertility. The same thing can happen with chlamydia, which has similar symptoms and consequences.

Genital herpes is a sexually transmitted viral infection. It is characterized by the appearance of small blisters on the genitals that in two or three days break and produce small, very painful sores. These lesions scar spontaneously in a few days, but they are never cured. In addition to contributing to an increased risk of cancer in the neck of the uterus, this infection can be transmitted to the child during delivery. You should be aware of this fact: this is considered one of the most frequently transmitted sexual diseases in the world.

There are other microorganisms which produce vaginal infections in women very frequently. The most common of these are Candida albicans (which produces moniliasis, commonly known as a yeast infection), trichomoniasis, and Gardnerella. The fundamental way these are transmitted is sexually, and especially the last two, if they are not addressed and treated promptly, can lead to a condition called vulvovaginitis, an inflammation of the vulva and the vagina and eventually to a pelvic inflammation in women with the further risk of ectopic pregnancy and sterility.

Vulvovaginitis presents as a burning in the vulva, discomfort upon urination, intense itching, and secretions with varied characteristics, according to which germ provoked it. In men, it generally does not produce any symptoms, but sometimes it can present as discomfort or burning upon urinating with local irritation.

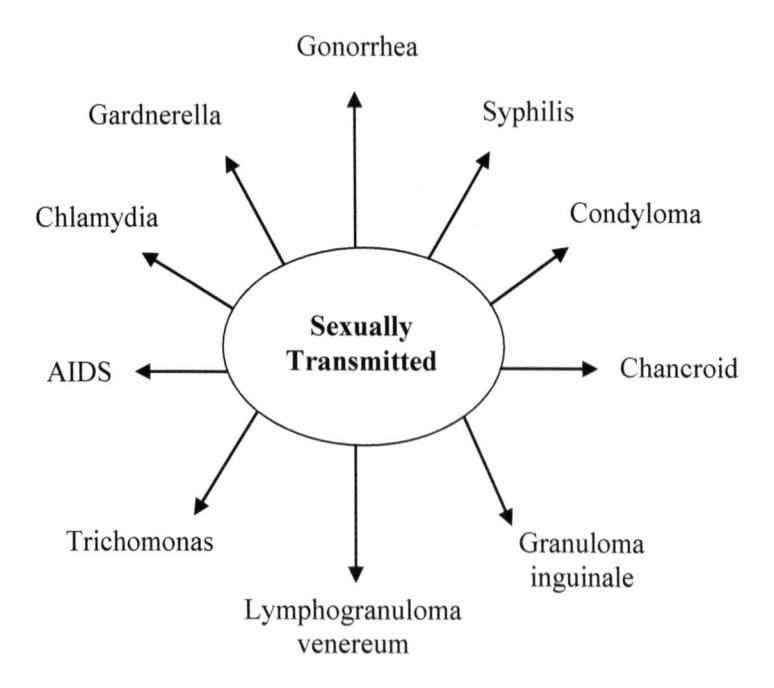

```
                    Gonorrhea
    Gardnerella              Syphilis

 Chlamydia                        Condyloma

                  ┌─────────────┐
                  │  Sexually   │
  AIDS   ←────────│ Transmitted │────────→ Chancroid
                  └─────────────┘

                                    Granuloma
    Trichomonas                     inguinale

                 Lymphogranuloma
                    venereum
```

These are some examples —only some— of infections that are transmitted primarily by sexual intercourse, since no less than twenty-five microorganisms and approximately fifty diseases that can be transmitted in this way have been identified to this day.

The most dangerous thing is that many times these infections are not detected, so that someone may seem like the healthiest person in the world yet suffer from one of these diseases. Another important thing: anyone can be infected, and, therefore, anyone can transmit them. In this matter, neither age, sex, race, nor vaccination count for anything. Any one of us could be affected! On the other hand, none of them produces immunity. With chickenpox, for example, once people have had it, they can be in contact with others who are sick with it and not be infected again. In the case of sexually transmitted diseases, exactly the opposite happens: those who have had one infection, whichever one, run a much greater risk of contracting the same one, or any other, again.

Now I am going to tell you something that you probably do not know: according to research that has been done on this subject, two out of three sexually transmitted infections occur in adolescents.

People who have the highest possibility to contract any sexually transmitted infection are those who change partners frequently and those who elect to have sex with someone they have just met without knowing what their new partner's sexual activity and habits have been or if they are promiscuous —that is, without knowing if they have had sexual intercourse with several people in a short period of time.

In adolescence, it is normal to change partners, because it is a time when we are looking for the right person with whom to have a long-lasting relationship. However, it is not good to have a new partner every week either; some adolescents, especially boys, sometimes change partners like they change their shirts, which turns into very risky sexual behavior, not only because they can easily be infected, but also because they can easily spread the infection to many others.

Here is something that should be taken into account: as a general rule, sexually transmitted diseases have worse consequences for women than for men. This is due to the characteristics of women's genital organs, which in addition to being more prone to infections, make diagnosis more difficult, since some of these diseases rarely show symptoms in the beginning stages, and when the lesions do appear, if the vagina and the neck of the uterus are not explored with a speculum, many times the infections can go undetected and continue to develop. This is why prevention continues to be the only effective weapon against these infections.

In this case, prevention = intelligence, because you should have sufficient intelligence not to initiate sexual intercourse until the required conditions exist for an act of love as important as this.

Once you have begun, you should seriously consider the following recommendations with the objective of reducing the risk of contamination to a minimum:

- Have sexual intercourse with one stable partner
- Be mutually faithful —that is to say, do not have casual sex with other partners
- Avoid promiscuity
- Do not have sexual intercourse with promiscuous people

Most important of all: ALWAYS USE A CONDOM, highlighted in capital letters so you do not forget, because it continues to be the most effective measure of prevention for preventing STDs. Condoms are available to everyone and always offer assurance to those who use them.

Like you have probably noticed, many microorganisms are ready and waiting for the first opportunity to do their thing and complicate our lives with a good number of diseases, threatening infertility and even leading to death. The weapons to prevent this are in your hands!

YOUR FRIEND THE GYNECOLOGIST

Your relationship with the gynecologist begins from the very moment you are born: he is the one who welcomes you to the world, receives your cries with joy, and is happy to see the smile on your parents' faces when they discover you. This relationship should be maintained for a lifetime, because girls as well as boys will need us many times.

Boys too? I really did not make a mistake when I wrote the previous paragraph. It is true that the gynecologist cares directly for women, but because we take care of girls and adolescents, we also receive the boys in our office. It is always better when the young woman comes in with her boyfriend or one of her close male friends from her group. This is the time when many of the worries that I have reflected upon on the pages of this book begin to show up, along with other fears that technically are of interest to the boys as well. I am a gynecologist, and I wrote this for the boys too.

Now that adolescence is here, it is time that you paid us a visit with any doubts or worries that you may have, without waiting until it is too late, after something has already happened. When it comes to gynecological matters and sexuality, we would rather offer guidance to young people early on, when they want to ask about some menstrual disorder, contraception, or any other related issue. This is better than later, after they arrive at the real worry of a pregnancy they did not expect or come in with an infection they never imagined they would have. With the passage of the years, when the time for pregnancy has come, you will return to our office —again, both of you— so that everything will turn out all right. Later, you will return again for a Pap smear or a simple breast exam, to avoid diseases, which appear during those years. I say both of you because men should not leave their partners alone during these moments.

A lot of doctors who work in outpatient clinics and hospitals find that patients come for a visit only when they are sick, but our patients visit us all their lives, and we are always ready to help any time they need us.

Your friend, the gynecologist, is always waiting for you.

EPILOGUE

I have attempted to help you. I do not know if I have achieved that goal, but at least I tried. Each of the subjects discussed in this book is an answer to some worry or other expressed by adolescents, including my daughters, who were adolescents when the inspiration for this book appeared and who were my primary editors when I was writing it. They were a great help when it came to finding out what the most important doubts were during this time of life.

It is difficult to summarize everything in just a few pages, but now after reading about the different parts, you already have a more complete idea about this subject, and surely you are ready to share your new knowledge with your friends. If you learned something new, if you agree with me about the different issues I discussed, and most of all, if you can follow the recommendations I made about sexual activity and its risk, then you and I can both feel very satisfied about the existence of this book.

Printed in Great Britain
by Amazon